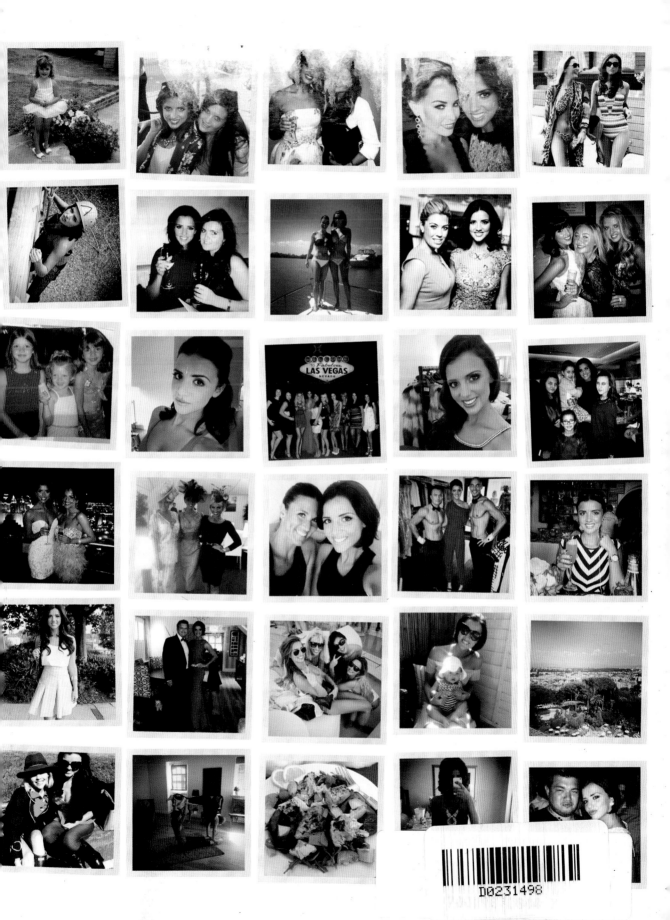

This book is dedicated to all the girls who have trusted me to help them transform their bodies – you are my inspiration! X

BE BODY BEAUTIFUL

MY GUIDE TO A HEALTHY, HAPPY NEW YOU

•

LUCY MECKLENBURGH

MICHAEL JOSEPH
an imprint of
PENGUIN BOOKS

MICHAEL JOSEPH

UK | USA | Canada | Ireland | Australia
India | New Zealand | South Africa

Michael Joseph is part of the Penguin Random House group
of companies whose addresses can be found at
global.penguinrandomhouse.com.

Penguin
Random House
UK

First published 2015
002

Text copyright © Lucy
Photography copyrigh
and Isabella Haigh, 20
Additional photograp
please see page 284 fo

Food styling by Hanna

The moral right of the

Designed by Smith & Gilmour
Set in 11.5/16pt Archer and Modern Extended
Colour reproduction by Alta Image
Printed and bound in Italy by Printer Trento s.r.l

A CIP catalogue record for this book is available from the British Library

ISBN: 978-0-718-18093-5

www.greenpenguin.co.uk

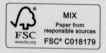

MIX
Paper from
responsible sources
FSC® C018179

Penguin Random House is committed to a
sustainable future for our business, our readers
and our planet. This book is made from Forest
Stewardship Council® certified paper.

Contents

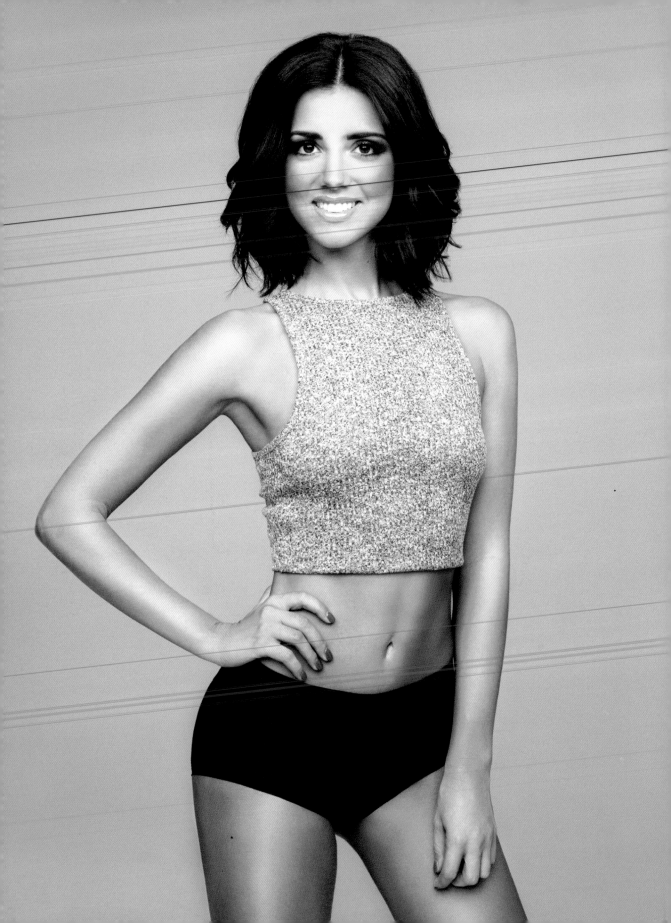

MY JOURNEY

I'm probably the happiest and most content I've ever been in my life at the moment. I don't think I've ever before been able to honestly say that I am totally happy with every part of my life but, right now, that's exactly what I am. It's a nice place to be.

I know how it feels to be unhappy in lots of ways, in particular about my body, but I also know how it feels to have worked really hard and transformed my body and my shape. This book is not only a personal journey I want to share with you but also, I'd like to hope, a useful tool that will help you feel body beautiful. I will share with you some of the secrets, techniques, tips and lifestyle changes that I use to make me feel as body confident as possible. No one should feel unhappy with their body because I strongly believe that we all have the power to change. Take control and get healthy – you have everything you need in this book to make it happen. I don't want excuses – we are all busy but you NEED to find the time to make the difference and, besides, this book is designed to be incorporated into hectic schedules. Make the change like me and you'll see the difference in every aspect of your life. I know I have.

'I NEVER THOUGHT
I COULD LOSE WEIGHT
AS EASILY AS THIS.'

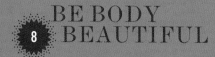

IN THE SPOTLIGHT

I'm finally happy with my weight. I'm healthy and, instead of fluctuating from curvy to skinny, I now stay at my 'me' weight and size. This hasn't been an easy road – especially as I've lived the most recent and influential parts of my life in front of a camera. My own choice, I know – but it has come with pressures I didn't realize even existed. Despite the pressures and difficulties, for the first time I can say that I feel confident and proud of myself. When I look in the mirror I am happy with the person who looks back at me, rather than thinking, 'I need to lose weight or I need to tone my bum.' Workwise, I am doing what I always dreamed of doing, and I'm in control of my life and where it's going, which just two years ago I would never have imagined myself being able to say. I have come a long way in that time. I have built a successful business – Results with Lucy and Lucy's Boutique – and in a way am giving something back to other people who feel the same way about their bodies as I used to.

Results with Lucy is a business built around people believing that they can achieve health and happiness no matter what their circumstances. Once that decision to get fit has been made, there's no excuse because my workouts are tailor-made for busy people and their lifestyles. It's changed people's lives … we are still changing people's lives.

'I FEEL I HAVE SO MUCH MORE SELF-CONFIDENCE AND ENERGY.'

Health and fitness is my addiction and my passion. I want to help others believe in themselves and believe that they can achieve whatever they want to in life. They just need to try. You just need to try. I can remember my dad saying to me, 'Lucy, just try your best and your best is all anyone can ask of you.' That's all anyone needs to do, their best.

In this book I want to tell you about how I've arrived at this point. How I became the girl that I am today. I don't want to be yet another celebrity that spills everything about their love life and takes shots at the various people they've fallen out with over the years to secure headlines. That's not what this is about. I want you to get to know me and who I really am. It's not always been easy – my parents divorced when I was eleven years old and I've had some pretty rocky relationships with boys, some of which many of you will be aware of … but I genuinely think that those experiences have made me stronger as a person and who I am today.

I was born in Brentwood in Essex and have always lived in that area – I still do! We moved a few times – Mum, Dad, my two sisters and me. I have one older sister called Christie and one younger sister called Lydia. But my mum (Linda) and my dad (Paul) split up when I was about nine years old and later divorced. I don't remember a lot about it because I was young. To be totally honest, I have blocked it out of my head. I don't want to remember it. There's really only one thing I do remember and that's packing my little sister Lydia's bag for her each time she went to stay with Dad. It used to really upset me that she was going, so I'd help her get ready and that way it didn't feel so sad for her to go away, more like it was an exciting trip instead. I think the family split affected my older sister more because she could properly understand what was going on.

Although I can't remember the details, it affected our life in material ways quite considerably. When we were a family unit we had quite a lot of money. Dad was earning well and we lived in a nice

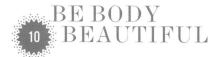

house in a nice area and we didn't want for anything. I laugh now because I only have about two designer items in my wardrobe but back then, literally, no word of a lie, my whole wardrobe was designer and that was the same for all of us. That's just how it was. But when Mum and Dad split up that had to change – they needed a house each and the money just wasn't there. I lived with my mum for three years before I decided, at the age of fourteen, that I wanted to change and live with my dad. It sounds like a big decision and in some ways I suppose it was, because I was leaving both my sisters and my mum behind and that was everything I had ever known, but in my mind I had a bedroom at my dad's house where I stayed twice a week anyway and it was the right thing to do, for me. More importantly, and perhaps the main reason for my decision, I was a real daddy's girl and I hated the idea of Dad being on his own. I moved in gradually, just staying with Dad more and more, so it wasn't like one day I was living at Mum's and the next I had packed up my room and moved to Dad's. I don't want to go into the details of that time but it all worked out and it was for the best.

At Mum's there were too many women under one roof for a start and the usual rows would happen between us all, over everything from sharing each other's clothes to nicking each other's make-up. We all clashed. My older sister was a swimmer and she wasn't really into the whole social scene like I was. She was happy to go to school and come home again and more or less do as she was told, but I was totally different from Christie and I'm not sure Mum knew how to deal with me. I was always trying to push the boundaries, like when I would sneak out to meet my mates or my boyfriend! I was a bit of a shock for her and she'd try to ground me or stop me doing something if I didn't behave or do what I was told. However, I needed to make my own mistakes and learn the hard way – even at that young age I knew it.

Every morning when my dad collected me to take me to school, my mum would chase me out of the house holding a facial wipe, trying to get me to take off all the make-up I'd put on. To be honest,

 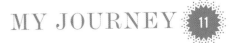

looking back, I was proper orange so she was right, but at the time there was no way I was going to do that! I used to wait until Mum went into the shower and then get Christie to iron my hair straight. I was strong-willed and it made for difficult living for all of us!

Dad was different. He got me a bit more and we have always been very close. Dad didn't have any rules really, which was very appealing at that age but it also made me independent and he allowed me to make my own mistakes, which I have learned from. If he did get cross with me he wouldn't speak to me for a few days and then he'd tell me that he was disappointed in me – which got me every time. I remember I once had a pool party at his house. He didn't know because he was out and I had to get everyone out of the house before 11 p.m. when he was coming back. Sam Faiers was there and we had a load of booze and one of the beer bottles managed to get lodged in the swimming pool filter! The next day Dad asked me if I had had a party the night before. I said, 'No.' He asked me again and told me it was the last time he'd ask the question but I said no again. And that was it. He didn't talk to me for days until I 'fessed up to the whole thing. He knew all along that I'd had the party but he wanted me to be honest about it. That was Dad's discipline system, but it worked for me – I needed that space to grow and make my own mistakes. That beer bottle cost him a fortune! One time I came home with a kitten called Cookie. Dad came back from work and saw this little ball of fluff. He was like, 'What is that?' His punishment for me was to keep the litter tray in my room!

The family break-up is probably quite significant in who I am today because it made me tougher. Choosing to live with my dad wasn't an easy decision but it made me quite hardy I guess. He doesn't show emotion; Dad was the kind of guy who would pat me on the back and say, 'You're all right, off you go.' He wouldn't embrace me or tell me that he loved me – that's not his style. I'm not complaining about that; in some ways I think it was a good way to have been brought up because I can pick myself up and brush

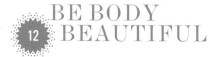

myself down and get on with things. He taught me that. However, I also know that my upbringing has had some bearing in that I can come across as quite cold. I find it hard to show emotions at times and I wish I didn't. We're just not really a family that says 'I love you' all the time – but we all know that we do.

While things were more laid back at Dad's, he and I didn't really know how or what to cook and eat. Most nights we would eat tomato sauce and pasta, pasta bolognaise or chilli con carne – in rotation. Mum had always been a great cook, cooking homemade meals and making sure that we ate healthily. She was quite strict about what we ate and there would never be any sweets in the cupboard or rubbish like that. She liked chocolate so there would always be a couple of chocolate bars hanging around but that was about it and when we came in after school we were only ever allowed to eat one snack so that we would eat all of our tea. Our tea would always have fresh vegetables or salad with it. I can remember going over to a school friend's house one time and being shocked that their mum ordered in six Domino's pizzas for us – a whole pizza each and we were only about nine years old! It was unbelievable and made me feel a bit sick. Even at that age I was aware that eating that sort of food was unhealthy and wasn't good for me. I think Mum had instilled that in us from an early age.

As I got older I inevitably fell into bad habits with food and drink. I binged like any other teenager does. I'd go on nights out and drink all the things that are totally horrendous for you like cheap rosé, vodka and Red Bull, Jägerbombs and sambuca. Seriously, it makes me feel sick when I think about it now! I really did like a drink . . . I suppose that's normal when you're young but although I still do like a drink I don't drink so excessively! It's quite scary how bad booze is for you and how many calories a glass of wine has. I mean it's fine to have occasionally, but you just need to be sensible about the limit and know when to stop. That's advice I could have done with a few years ago! One night I can remember drinking ten vodka and Red Bulls. I got home and I couldn't sleep all night because my heart was racing so much and I had to go to work the next day on no sleep. I felt

'I WANT YOU TO GET TO KNOW ME
        AND WHO I REALLY AM'

'I THINK THAT THOSE
         EXPERIENCES HAVE
    MADE ME STRONGER
AS A PERSON AND
        WHO I AM TODAY.'

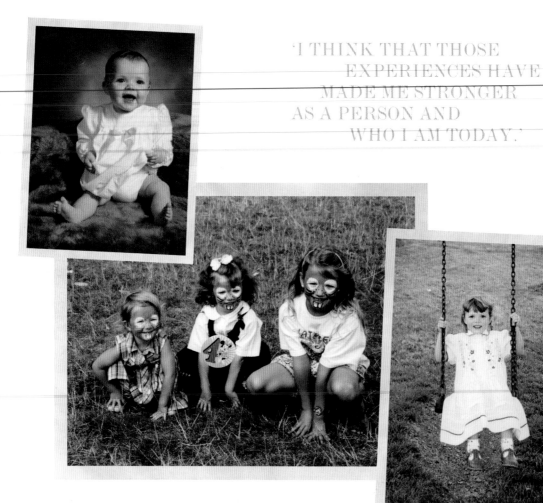

'THE FAMILY BREAK-UP IS
    PROBABLY QUITE SIGNIFICANT
IN WHO I AM TODAY BECAUSE
    IT MADE ME TOUGHER.'

'THERE'S REALLY ONLY ONE THING I DO
        REMEMBER [ABOUT MY PARENTS' DIVORCE]
    AND THAT'S PACKING MY LITTLE SISTER
            LYDIA'S BAG FOR HER EACH TIME
SHE WENT TO STAY WITH DAD.'

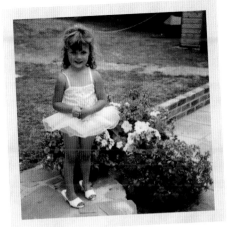

'I NEEDED TO MAKE MY
    OWN MISTAKES AND LEARN
THE HARD WAY – EVEN AT
    THAT YOUNG AGE I KNEW IT.'

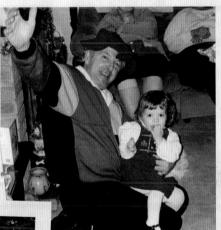

'I WAS A REAL DADDY'S GIRL
    AND I HATED THE IDEA
OF DAD BEING ON HIS OWN.'

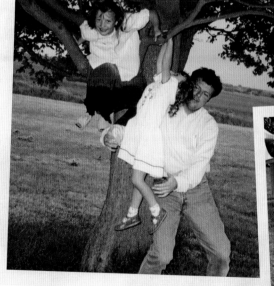

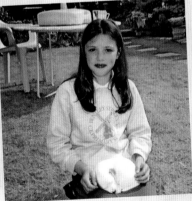

'IT'S NOT ALWAYS BEEN EASY –
    MY PARENTS DIVORCED WHEN
I WAS ELEVEN YEARS OLD AND
    I'VE HAD SOME PRETTY ROCKY
RELATIONSHIPS WITH BOYS'

totally rubbish. I'd get myself into all sorts of situations and the amount of times I had to sneak back home by climbing in through my bedroom window I can't count on just two hands. Luckily Dad had a bungalow! Half the time I'm sure he thought I was tucked up in bed, really I was sneaking out of the window, going out for the night and only getting back before it was light. Sorry, Dad. But I did know that sometimes he was sneaking in at 4 a.m. after me! He's a real party animal. These days if I want to go out on a Friday I'll text my dad and see if he wants to go out with me. On the night we finished filming *Tumble*, he came out with all of us and we ended up in Soho for breakfast. He texted me the next day and said, 'If I lived in London, I'd be dead!'

These days my naughty drink is a Bellini. I only have one to start the night off with and then I move on to vodka and soda with fresh lime. That is literally my favourite drink ever. And at dinner I'll have a nice glass of Rioja. I love red wine. I have learned that it is all about moderation.

When I was younger I don't think I even knew what moderation meant . . . I'd drink while I was getting ready to go out with my mates and then when I actually got out I would drink a fair bit more and then grab a burger or kebab on the way home – that's just what you do when you're growing up. I never let things get too out of hand but my body was changing and I wasn't entirely happy with what I saw looking back at me in the mirror. Weight can literally just fall off me and looking back I can see a clear pattern in my yo-yoing weight and body shape. It's not a healthy way to be and by fluctuating like that your body never really knows where it stands.

Excesses in life take a massive toll on your skin and energy levels and I think your positivity and drive disappear when you get like that. Now that I have a good understanding of nutrition and what my body needs, choosing a kebab seems completely alien to me. I can't even imagine ordering one let alone eating it. Yuck. When I lived at my dad's, there was a 24-hour McDonalds nearby and I'd have a burger every day. Gross.

BE BODY
BEAUTIFUL

There were two real turning points for me to decide to get fit. The first was when I went to buy a new pair of jeans – it was when Mario and I were dating. Growing up I was always a size 6–8 but I knew my weight had been creeping up. I took a size 10 into the changing rooms and I couldn't get them on. The fitting-room assistant asked me if she could get me a size 12. I felt horrible – I was like, 'NO WAY!' – and I literally ran out of the shop. I was so upset at how I'd changed that I cried. I'm not for a minute saying that a size 12 is big, I'm really not. It's just that it was too big for me and my height.

A few days later, Mario and I went to Mexico on holiday. The paparazzi managed to find out where we were staying and spent the day taking photos of us, but we had no idea. Then I saw the pictures: of me stuffing my face, in a bikini and generally looking really awful, printed in magazines and newspapers. I was so embarrassed, it crushed me. I thought that I looked fat and horrible. I felt sick even just looking at the pictures because Mario was very toned and buff. He took real care of his appearance whereas I felt I looked really bad in comparison. Everything was going through my mind, wondering if I could stop the photos from being published anywhere ever again, but that wasn't an option.

Being completely honest, those Mexico pictures devastated me. I know that might sound dramatic but when you read nasty things about your body it's a horrible feeling. Up until that point I hadn't been used to that. I'd never really considered that my body was in bad shape but after the jeans incident and then, when I looked at those pictures, it was a massive reality check. The issue wasn't even about size for me, it was about my health. I wasn't being healthy with my diet and in turn I was tired, emotional and my skin was getting pimply. The pressure of my life being played out on a reality show was really getting to me; plus Mario and I were just starting to go through a difficult patch. When I get very low, weight tends to drop off, as I said, but this was that in-between stage when I was still relatively content in my relationship, although problems were afoot, and my life was getting on top of me. Looking back I can see that

I wasn't happy and clearly it was showing in my body. I looked puffy, I wasn't toned and I had cellulite. For the first time I had cellulite and it really got to me. I was miserable and I was generally eating terrible food. I was a mess. Every comment I read on the Internet seemed to agree with me! I saw comments like: 'There is nothing toned about her whatsoever,' and 'She needs to work on her bum.' It was awful and embarrassing. The pictures were everywhere and it gave me a literal kick up the arse to do something about my situation. So, when I got home from Mexico, that's when I decided I was going to get fit, strong and healthy. By nature I'm pretty disciplined but I have always, for as long as I can remember, HATED the gym . . .

I know lots of people will think I'm being ridiculous or that it's wrong of me to feel like I do about those pictures or about being a size 12. I'm just being really honest about how I felt. A size 12 was not right for me. That's part of my message – you have to do what is right for your body. I am not comfortable at that size. I didn't feel healthy and I wanted to change for me – that was not my 'happy weight' if you like. I needed to do something because it was getting me down and those pictures were the push I needed to start exercising and looking at what I ate.

I knew at the time that I was in a real slump and that deep down I wanted to make a change but like I said – when I am content I tend to eat. I get comfortable quite quickly and Mario and I would go out for lots of lovely meals. Or I'd wait at home for him to come back from work and then we'd order a takeaway. It was obvious that the weight was going to creep on. It wasn't a healthy, balanced lifestyle that we were leading and that was why I was up two dress sizes. I think every individual knows when they start to get overweight and feel uncomfortable and I had got to that point. My confidence was low and I started to cover myself up. I wasn't proud of the way I looked and I didn't want anyone to see me. This was a new feeling for me and I didn't like it one bit. I'd always been pretty outgoing and confident with my body shape. I hated that I wanted to wear longer shorts or skirts because I was embarrassed by the way

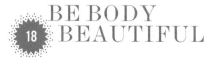

I looked. Mario never said anything about me being overweight – in fact, I doubt he thought I was – but I knew I wanted to change. Not for anyone else, just for me.

Like everyone, over the years I'd tried all sorts of different exercise regimes. I'd previously bought an annual gym membership but I think I managed to motivate myself to get down there just twice and when I did go the gym looked really daunting and I can remember thinking, 'Where on earth do I start?' That was the point when I went home again! No workout done and a heap of money spent that I could have put towards a pair of Louboutins!

When I started my business I wanted to provide a practical way of helping people incorporate exercise and healthy eating into their busy lives. I reached a point where I was unhappy with my body and wanted to do something about it, but I wanted a fun, flexible routine, not something else to feel guilty about. Results with Lucy employs over thirty people now and basically what we do is create films of different workouts and design daily meal plans that the people who have subscribed to the website can follow. We have a whole team of skilled videographers for the filming process. There are loads of different workouts in the programme now – about three hundred in total – and we have grown each year to be bigger and better, offering more and more to our subscribers. In the beginning it was just myself, Cecilia Harris and her husband Frank. I met Cecilia when I first started to train in 2013 and we became friends and then business partners. The idea was born from when we were training together: Cecilia would take a picture of me and post it on Twitter. SO MANY people started asking how to train like me that we thought: let's do this. Let's turn this idea into reality and start a business, and that's what we did. It's not just us any more either – we employ yoga, ballet and Pilates teachers. We also have a guy called Liam Willis who specializes in posture and movement, which often helps those who are suffering with a bad back or problems with their joints or even digestion. These sorts of physical issues can stop people from being able to exercise and work out as they want to or should be able to. The idea of having so many different people on board at Results with Lucy was so that we could offer all sorts of different styles of training. Each person has a preferred method of exercise and we can provide all of those different possibilities – which is really exciting and, most importantly, it is totally affordable. We have a YouTube channel for Results with Lucy and on there we record a lot of the different workouts too and that gives people an idea of what we have to offer and what we can do for them.

When Cecilia, Frank and I first started, I was prepared for the whole business start-up thing to be really hard. I thought it was such a competitive market but, without sounding too smug, it's just gone from strength to strength, right from the moment we started. We've been incredibly lucky but, at the same time, when we came up with the idea we knew there wasn't anyone else really offering what we wanted to do. The closest match to what we were thinking of was happening in the US and, when we looked at their workouts and philosophies, we thought, 'We could do this so much better.' We 100% believed in our idea, our plan of action and our goals, and I think that positivity really helped our success. Within two weeks we had already covered our start-up costs and we were making a profit within a month. It was quite astonishing and proved that there's a huge market for what we offer.

At first I had thought about doing a fitness DVD – a bit like every other celebrity does – but I wanted to be credible and I wanted to be taken seriously. Most fitness DVDs work from the person being overweight then losing the weight, only to put it back on again and lose it again. That's a totally unhealthy cycle and goes against everything I believe in, so I knew making a fitness DVD wasn't for me. I think most DVDs end up collecting dust on your shelf after two months! This online workouts idea seemed to be the perfect solution and it's been amazing. The more people liked it, the better we did and the more confident we became in the product we were offering. Results with Lucy was genuinely turning people's lives around, and still does.

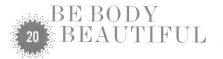

When we first started I didn't really know what I was doing. I had experience of retail sales and was running my own boutique – Lucy's Boutique – so I knew all about fashion retail but nothing about the fitness industry. It was a huge learning curve for me. Before *TOWIE*, I was working as a showroom model and in sales for Forever Unique (a clothing company) and I had no real idea at all about running my own business. We literally started from scratch, found ourselves an office in Essex and that's where we still are today! Our success is proof that, if nothing else, when you have a dream you should go for it. If I can do it, so can you.

All our workouts are recorded by our film crew and usually involve me being trained by Cecilia. We think it's really important to give each subscriber a personal touch. I think it encourages whoever they are to really get stuck in and do well. They know we are there if they run into any trouble or if they have a day when they don't want to do something and need a little encouragement. Our feeling was, and still is, that people get fed up with hefty gym memberships and this offers an alternative to that. Over 50,000 girls have taken up the Results with Lucy programme, which is an absolute dream. I still sometimes wake up and pinch myself. To know that we are helping that many people is amazing. It's an incredible feeling to be able to help people and touch their lives and know that we really are boosting women's confidence.

Now we have almost every workout imaginable available to our users. Last August we launched Results with Bump – after many of our subscribers became pregnant and wanted to keep working out – which has been a huge success already. For a lot of women, when they get pregnant they think that it signals the end of their body shape and they resign themselves to the idea that they will never get it back, but that doesn't need to be the case. There are really sensible workouts for expectant mums to do to keep themselves healthy while they are pregnant. Not only is it good for mum but it is also good for baby. Once the baby has been born we provide workouts to ease the mums back into doing some light exercise and at their

 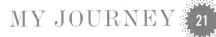

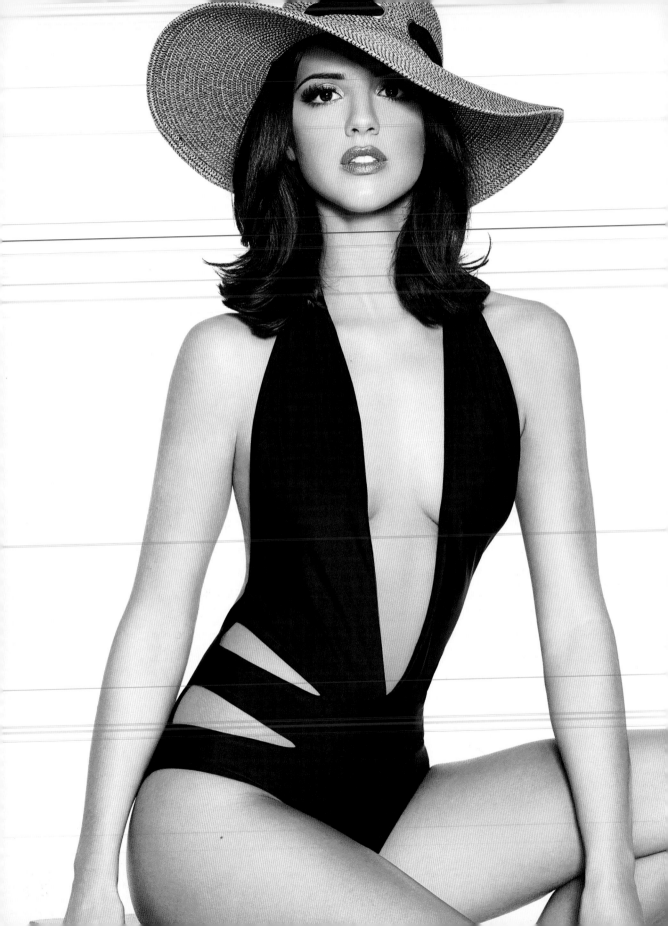

own pace. When you have a new baby, time is precious and you are very tired and we take all of those things into account. Because I've never had a baby I got Claire Sweeney involved. She is the brand ambassador for it and has filmed a lot of the workouts. I didn't feel in a position to advise new and expectant mums, not having gone through that experience myself, but I knew that I wanted to help people who were asking me how to exercise when pregnant and train afterwards too.

In the past I had tried a couple of boot camps and I'd hated them. They were full of military instructors who shouted and screamed and generally made me feel awful. You're fed virtually nothing and you are pushed to your limit until you are physically sick. It's exhausting and completely unsustainable. I felt not only physically drained but also emotionally drained by the end. I can remember on one boot camp I lost 7 pounds and 7 inches in a week. At that time I was only a size 8 so I couldn't really afford to lose that much weight, but that wasn't taken into consideration – it was simply a boot camp that ran you ragged.

Cecilia and I got talking about this and thought there must be a way of running a boot camp that is enjoyable and sustainable. Where you get something out of it for the long term as well as the short term. We started by writing down all the things we hated about boot camps and then working out how we could offer something totally different. Our 'bootycamps' aren't a breeze, but many women who attend do come back again and that says a lot, I think, for what the experience is like. How many women do you know who want to roll in mud all weekend to lose a few pounds? And in winter – why make people train outside in the freezing cold? It's ridiculous. If they have to be up at 6am, the last thing they want to do is go outside in the freezing cold. These military-style boot camps make training as unappealing as possible, I think! Our programme is much more enjoyable.

We don't just focus on exercise – although that's obviously key – as we have supportive instructors who understand that training and pushing your body is hard and some people won't have exercised for years. They're not there to get shouted at by us, they are there to be encouraged and motivated to continue once the bootycamp is over. One aspect that is massively popular is our mixture of exercise classes with burlesque classes and yoga. Then in the evenings we offer massages for people and their aching limbs! There are no other boot camps quite like ours and they've proved to be massively popular.

At some point during the camp, I always go and give a talk so that people can understand our philosophy and why health and exercise is so important. In many ways, although there are a lot of calories burned over the weekend, it's really about re-educating people about food. I hear so many people say, 'I can't lose weight and I don't know why. I don't eat breakfast and I skip lunch but I can't shift the pounds.' That's easy to explain because they have answered their own question. It's because they aren't eating breakfast or lunch that they are overweight. There's a saying that fat people don't eat breakfast and it's true. It's key to a healthy eating plan and on the bootycamp weekends I explain to people why certain meals are so important – for example, breakfast. It kick-starts your metabolism for the day and it stops you having that mid-morning slump when you want to grab a chocolate bar.

It became clear to us that we needed to employ a nutritionist at Results with Lucy to give our subscribers the added benefit of meal plans in combination with our workouts. We are a nation of clueless people when it comes to nutrition and there are so many mixed messages on the supermarket shelf. Cecilia knew Emma Whitnall, an amazing nutritionist coach, and so she joined the team. In the same way that Cecilia started out as my personal trainer, now Emma also works with me as my personal nutritionist. On the Saturday night at our bootycamps she gives a motivational nutrition talk. She talks about relationships with food and answers a lot of questions for people. I think her talk is often the most popular part of the weekend because it includes so many surprising facts.

I don't think anyone can believe how much they are allowed to eat over the weekend – but always the right stuff. It's often been said by people on our bootycamps that they have never eaten so much and

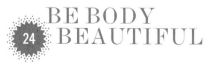

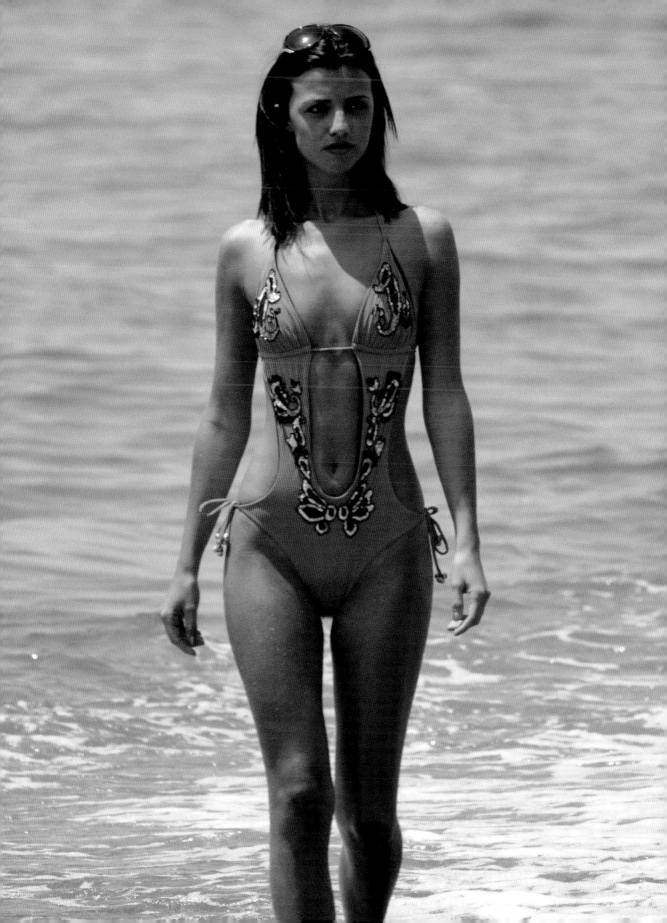

still lost weight, and that's the proof that if you eat well you don't need to feel hungry. Those mid-afternoon chocolate bars that give you an instant sugar rush and wake you up are such a short-term fix because within an hour your body will be low again. If you don't eat processed food and follow a really healthy, balanced meal plan, you will almost instantly feel better. By following the meal planners in this book you WILL:

1 Gain energy.

2 Your skin will look brighter and, perhaps, most importantly...

3 You will start to lose weight.

At the end of Emma's nutrition talk we have a question and answer session with myself, Emma and Cecilia and we answer, within reason, what anyone wants to know! This is extremely popular with people and therefore I am thinking about starting to run nutrition seminars. It's a topic that many people really are uneducated about. They will often just look at the number of calories and decide on their lunch based on that, when there are so many other factors to take into account. I truly believe that once you have made the change and you understand food then you will never go back to your old eating habits.

Before I became so passionate about exercise and found ways to actually enjoy it, the whole process was a massive effort and I just couldn't find something that suited me. I think that's a problem for a lot of people. You know you want to make a change and to exercise but fundamentally don't know where to start.

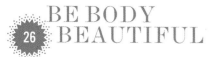

I feel like I can speak with experience on this subject because not only have I been too big (in my opinion) but I've also been too thin. I think some people fail to recognize when they get too small. They get carried away by feeling good in themselves and when people say things like, 'Wow – you've lost a lot of weight,' it almost spurs them on to lose even more. The less you eat the less you want to eat and that's not a good cycle to get into. At the end of my relationship with Mario, I was unhappy and I had no appetite, and so I lost a lot of weight. Too much weight. At one point I was barely a size 6. In US terms that basically made me a size zero. I'm not proud of that and, when I look at pictures from that time, I realize how unhealthy I had become. If you see the pictures of me in Marbella with the other girls in 2013 I am literally half their size – or less – and in the *TOWIE* calendar shoot in May that year I look tiny by comparison. I know it wasn't a healthy way to be but at that point it hadn't really dawned on me how small I really was. I didn't see what other people were seeing. I was wrapped up in my own feelings and emotions after my break-up with Mario. I was feeling low and in a rut and I didn't have the inclination to take care of myself. Yes, I was exercising and I still had energy but that's not everything that's needed to be healthy.

I can remember going on a shoot for *Hello!* magazine. The stylist gave me a pink Zara jumpsuit to wear, which I loved because just a couple of days earlier I had bought one myself although I hadn't actually tried it on. The stylist got me an extra-small size and it literally fell off me. She looked at me and said, quite seriously, 'Lucy, you need to put on some weight.' I remember thinking that if a stylist thinks I'm too thin I really must be – they work with tiny models all of the time, yet she still thought I was too skinny. I looked again in the mirror and I looked really hard and what I saw was a woman without any curve to her. All my womanly curves had disappeared and I don't think any man would say that was very sexy or attractive. I knew I needed to do something to get my body to the best healthy place that I could and to stick to it. I knew then that I didn't want to spend my life fluctuating from one extreme to the other.

After the break-up with Mario, my addiction had become exercise. Instead of turning to something unhealthy that gave me a short-term fix, for once I did the right thing but – like I often do – I went too far. I know the problem was my mental state rather than my working out and I had to start to reign myself back in. I don't think people realize that being thin can be as bad as being overweight. As I understand it, the US has the highest statistics when it comes to clinically obese people and I don't think the UK is far behind. Obviously that's not a good place to be – it can lead to all sorts of health problems like heart disease or diabetes – but, because of that, we all focus on being slimmer and healthier. However that can go too far, and I'm an example of it. Being underweight has its own issues.

At some point I want to have a family and I don't want to jeopardize that by doing something silly that wrecks my body for the future. Being too thin can often affect fertility – sometimes your periods can stop and it can affect your hormones, which in turn affect your chances of conceiving. I know that I need to be in control rather than my body ever being in control of me. To let your weight have that level of control over you is madness. I was buying clothes that were a size 4 and I know that's too small. Articles were being written in the press about me being too thin and, in the same way that it's not nice reading people say that you are too fat, it's also not nice to read the opposite. I don't want to hear people calling me a 'skinny bitch' or saying that I am 'bony'. When that started happening it was horrible. Not just for me, but my family too. They could see that I had lost a lot of weight and, if I'm totally truthful, there were two schools of thought. My sisters knew I'd lost weight but thought I still looked good; they certainly didn't think that I was wasting away. And I wasn't. Yes, I was gaunt and yes, I was much smaller then I probably should have been but I was a long way from 'ill' thin. One thing I will admit, though, is that being thinner got me a lot of attention. I am not an attention-seeker, I'm not looking to make headlines or to try and feel better about myself that way, but I had a glimpse of how and why people might go too far.

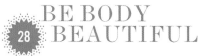

By losing weight you often get more attention, but it's for the wrong reasons.

Weight is a very personal matter and you have to deal with it in your own way and in your own time. Outside pressure doesn't help the situation, so if my family or friends had been on at me then it probably would have made things worse. Sometimes you shut down when people keep on and I'm quite stubborn. If I'd had a load of people in my ear about my weight it would have probably just wound me up rather than doing anything positive. My mum said a few things to me but that's what mums do, isn't it? One time – when I was over at my mum's, when I hadn't seen her for a little while – she took one look at me and said, 'Lucy, you're wasting away.' She wasn't happy with how I looked and she thought I should put on some weight. She told me to slow down with my training because I think she blamed that for my weight loss, but really I was being strict with myself over everything. Mum cooked dinner and then afterwards she tried to force me to eat dessert! It was her way of trying to help! What I didn't realize is that Mum was very like me when she was younger and her weight fluctuated too. When she gets worried or stressed, the weight just falls off her. For instance, when she got married to my dad she was really stressed and nervous and she lost so much weight that her dress had to be taken in. She was tiny.

I'm not suggesting for a minute that I had an eating disorder because I didn't. I want to make that absolutely clear now because while I am being completely open about how I feel about my weight and how I have felt about it over the years, I have never made myself sick to lose weight or been anorexic. I'm pretty sure that my honesty reflects what most girls feel about themselves if they were to tell the

'I KNOW THAT I NEED TO BE IN CONTROL RATHER THAN MY BODY BEING IN CONTROL OF ME.'

 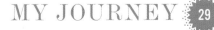

absolute truth. But, at that time, I was being really strict with my eating and I was doing a lot of exercise. I was unhappy and it was a bad combination.

There's also something else that played on my mind and I don't think you can underestimate the effect that boys have on girls. I've always been proud of the fact that I am strong-minded, but boys have this weird way of getting into your head and you do care what they think. Mario had always been very complimentary about my body but one night we were getting ready for bed and I could see him looking at me. He told me that I had the body of an eleven-year-old boy. I used to have pert, larger boobs and through the weight loss I had lost them. I was looking flatter than I ever had before. It was a horrible moment and what he said really hurt me. It stuck with me for a long time and I couldn't get it out of my head. I kept thinking I've lost my curves and I need to get them back.

Now I am a healthy size 8 and it's pretty much a case of maintenance. Of course, I still get a bashing from the press at times about my weight and people say that I am too thin but I'm not – I am at a healthy weight and I know how to keep it relatively static. I went on a ski trip earlier this year and, since I was on holiday, of course I was eating like you do when you are on holiday, and I put on some weight. So, when I got back I did some juicing to lose the extra pounds. It was a healthy way of knocking the excess weight off. Emma always recommends a three-day juicing detox programme. Some people do it for longer but it's been suggested that that can slow your metabolism down. I don't want to lose any weight – I just want to make sure that I stay like I am because, as I mentioned earlier, I am at my happy weight. I'm not too thin and I'm not too big. This is my right size. Once you are where you want to be you need to recognize that and maintain it. That's the key to loving your body and keeping it healthy – re-educating the way you think because very often what you see in the mirror is not what other people see

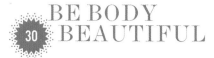

and that can be very dangerous. A distortion of reality. Mario, rightly or wrongly, telling me that I had the body of an eleven-year-old is a good example of that. Perhaps I had a distorted view of myself…

Most recently I have taken part in *Tumble* on BBC1. I'll tell you more about the show later but the gymnastic training I had to undertake has really changed my body shape. I started to get a bum for the first time and I really love it! I'm not saying I want a Kim Kardashian arse but I do want to try and keep the shape of my new bum because it gives me some womanly curves. If there's one thing I've learned (and not just from Mario!) it's that men do like a curvy lady. Straight up and down isn't the best look. Even though the training has now stopped I am going to try and incorporate some aspects of it into a few new workouts on my website so other people can get a bum like that too!

For me, getting healthy is the best thing I have ever done. I can honestly say that. I have taken control of 'me' and I know what is right for my own body. Identifying it was all part of the battle. Once your attitude changes towards both exercise and food there is no going back. I am energized and I feel more confident than ever. It's a life change. If you follow this book's advice you will look and feel great. And remember: DON'T feel guilty if you do have a chocolate bar or a packet of crisps. Move on, it's a new day and a fresh start. I have written easy-to-follow meal planners, as well as exercise plans, to help everyone achieve their long-term goals. Remember my motto: 'A healthy body, a happy you.' Stick with this programme and you can achieve the body of your dreams. It'll be tough at times and there will be moments you want to throw the towel in – I know I did. But I promise that if you hold on in there and put in the effort, it really works. That old saying 'No pain, no gain' is true but don't make a big thing of it. This is a change you have already decided to embark on. Believe in yourself and in no time at all a new person will be staring back at you in the mirror and you'll LOVE it! That alone makes it all worthwhile.

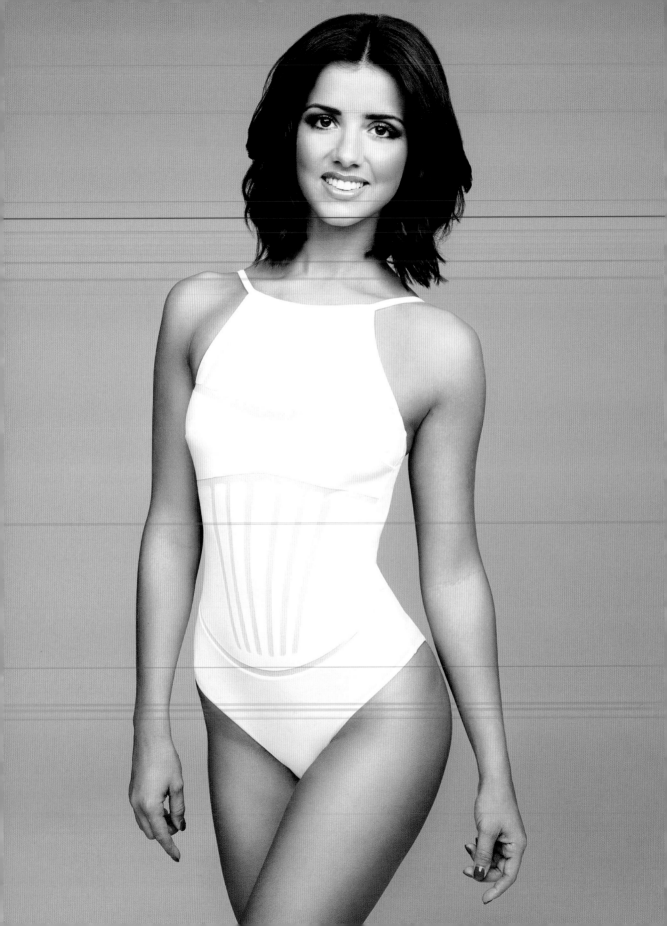

2
MOTIVATE

There comes a point in most people's lives that makes them sit up and think, 'I wanna change.' But making that change is the hardest part of all. Often the moment when you decide you want to change is a time when you aren't mentally at your strongest and that makes it even tougher. I know, because I speak from experience.

But, once you have made that decision to change, then stick with it. I turned to exercise and it made a huge difference to my mental state. After all, you need something to take your mind off the problem that's made you want to change in the first place! I sound like I'm talking in riddles but each person's reason for change will be unique. It might be a relationship, it might be a bereavement. It could be anything that signals that first trigger.

For me, exercise was the thing that turned my whole life around. It's become my best friend and now I couldn't live without it. Exercise provides so much that I need and has made me feel MUCH happier in myself. It can have that effect on you too, if you just give it a go. Scrap the excuses and the moaning and get out and do something active because it will make you happy.

I'm massively opinionated when it comes to health and exercise and I'm not afraid to say what I think. I don't have a good body because I sit about all day and eat. I have a good body because I eat well and I exercise. It's simple and that's why it annoys me SO much when people moan and whine about their weight or body yet do sweet FA about it. How many kids do you see that are too heavy? Too many. It's not their fault; it's the fault of the parents feeding them the crap in the first place. And don't get me started on plus-size ranges. You shouldn't need plus-size clothes – they are unhealthy. You shouldn't be that big and there is no reason to stay that big. I cannot understand why people endorse them as a good thing; it's beyond me. I'm not being fat-ist, I just want the world to be healthy and to make people realize that you can do something about it. Unless there are medical reasons why not, everyone can, they just need to put in a bit of time and willpower.

QUICK FIXES

We all want a quick fix but short of having lipo all over (which I wouldn't advocate!) there isn't a quick fix. The more hard work you put in, the sooner your body will start to take shape. In this book I have included a six-week plan including what to eat and what exercise to do and if you stick with it the results will be clear to see. Six weeks is pretty fast for a body overhaul.

I introduced exercise into my life before changing my diet and really the two go hand in hand. It wasn't until my diet also changed that I saw a completely different me. Change one thing at a time if you think that's easier but, long term, the only way to sustain a look is by balancing all of your life, including what you eat.

When you first start to think about exercise, work out what you enjoy. Cycling? Running? Swimming? It's far easier to choose something that you enjoy rather than making yourself do something that you hate. For years I tried forcing myself to go to the gym and I hated it. Running on the spot on a treadmill isn't for me so I had to find a way to replace the gym but get the same results. I have included some different routines for people wanting to exercise at home or in the park – sometimes these options are a lot less scary.

Variation in how you're working out will help make the biggest difference in a rapid journey to being healthy. When I started Results with Lucy, I really wanted to focus on lots of different exercises because who doesn't feel bored doing the same things over and over? Repetition soon gets boring and when you're bored you're not going to make ANY progress – let alone quick progress. I'd much rather be out with the girls than in the gym doing the same old stuff day after day. Not only that but as well as keeping you interested, a changing routine will give you faster and more visible results, like it did for me. Following a plan is really good – even if you're going to change the plan on a regular basis to keep it fresh – to make sure that you actually do SOMETHING!

'EXERCISE HAS
TURNED MY
WHOLE
LIFE AROUND.'

So that's my advice for getting a quick-fix body of your dreams. It's all about finding the balance between attitude, diet and exercise (plus throw in a bit of style and a bit of fake-tan, obvs!) and the fix you're after will be staring back at you when you look in the mirror.

MAKING EXERCISE A DAILY THING!

One of the biggest problems I had when I first began to take getting fit and healthy seriously was doing it on a regular basis. It's all fun and games when you start out. You've got some new selfies to upload on Instagram and it's all still a novelty. But that soon wears off. One way I combatted this was to get moving FIRST THING in the morning! This way I wasn't spending the whole day thinking up excuses to not have to work out and it was over and done with before I could moan to any of the girls. You feel pretty smug for the rest of the day too – knowing it's all in the bag.

The hard part is getting started because once it's in your routine it just feels normal. You'll soon be taking the stairs and not the lift – because your whole attitude to a healthy lifestyle will have changed. I feel guilty if I take the lift when I could be using the stairs now whereas at one time the idea of using the stairs wouldn't even have entered my head. Decisions like taking the stairs or a lift became no-brainers – and all these little things add up and start to make REAL differences in your fitness. Another one is parking the car in a far-away spot or just leaving it at home altogether – every step counts!

The main reason I think it was so easy to make exercising an everyday thing was because I avoided any major disruptions to my life. Unless you're a really strong person, making this massive turnaround in your life to get more active can be really hard when it really doesn't need to be! Make exercise and eating healthily part of your day. If you don't, you won't do it.

I think tracking your progress and planning for the future can be really helpful too if you want exercise every day. I remember when Mario and I had split but I was still on *TOWIE* and we had to film in Marbs. I knew that I had to be wearing a bikini and that I needed to look good, so that became my goal. I wanted my body fit and looking better than ever when I walked out in that white bikini. Put a goal in place and work towards it – that always helps with motivation. In the same way, if you know how far you've come in the last week, month, year then that will act as a huge motivation for you and really help to keep you going. It's all about reminding yourself why you're making this life change and, seriously, before you know it you won't remember your old ways of endless snacking and couch slumming.

'PUT A GOAL IN PLACE
AND WORK
TOWARDS IT.'

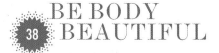

BE BODY
BEAUTIFUL

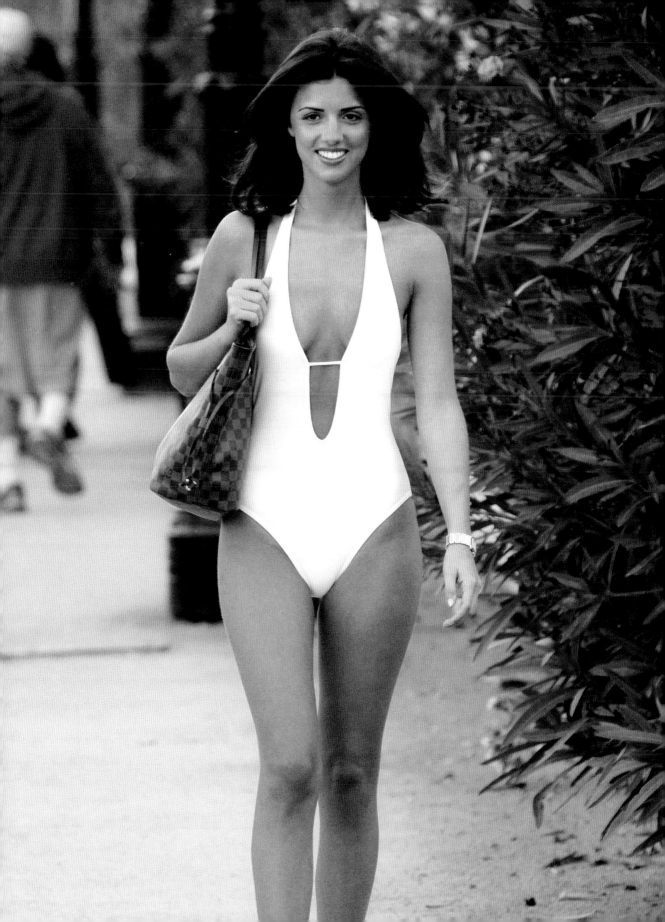

MAKING THE NEW YOU LAST A LIFETIME!

The key, I think, to making this process work is by making it your routine. Factor it into your day and prioritize it; don't let exercise be the thing that you do if you have time. If exercise becomes habitual then you've nailed it. Tailoring your workout so that it is perfect for you is probably my best advice to making sure you stick to it – who's going to keep doing something that they hate?

Another tip is to encourage your friends to join in. If you're all in the same boat then it'll be a lot more fun and you're more likely to carry on. A little competition between friends is really healthy for everyone's development, plus if a friend's going, you will want to go with them – it definitely helps morale. I'd be lying if I said there weren't times when I didn't want to get up, particularly at the very start, but when you have the girls encouraging you and reminding you of how important it is, you won't want to give up and let them down.

Keeping to this, making sure you don't skip a workout or start having more and more cheat days is REALLY important. There's nothing worse than seeing all of the progress you've made get thrown away like a cheap pair of eyelashes. This is something you have to stick to. Don't let cheat days become habit – if you don't have time for your full workout, try and just do as much of it as you can.

Remember it's ongoing! Everyone is a work in progress. Even if you're at what you feel is your perfect body, you need to keep going because maintaining that body is part of it all. You're never finished being healthy – it's a lifetime change. Your routine is something that you can change if it starts to feel like it isn't working for you, but why fix something that isn't broken? If you're going to change your routine, change it to something that will work for you this time and learn from your mistakes. Similar to making sure it's right for you, make sure that the exercise routine is at the right time for you and allows you to do it regularly, or else you'll find yourself quitting before you know it!

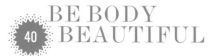

With something lasting as long as a lifetime it's so, so important to make sure that you enjoy it. There's no way you'll be able to keep something up that makes you sad and is a burden in your life; it's just not going to work. If that's the case, it's probably the workouts and routine that you're currently doing – not working out in general – that is the problem.

It doesn't matter how old you are, it's never too late to make the change. I think a lot of people think that they are too old and use that as an excuse as to why they don't start. Or people that have never worked out before worry that they don't know what they are doing or find the idea of going to a gym completely overwhelming. Busy mums will often complain that there is no time in their day to incorporate exercise, but there is. You just need to think about it and how you will start to incorporate it as part of your everyday life, not as an extra. From taking the stairs rather than the lift to parking your car at the supermarket in the spot furthest away from the shop so you have to walk further: it ALL helps. Excuses really do piss me off because that's all they are – an excuse not to make a change that will ultimately make you happier and healthier. Everyone can do it; you just have to want to.

Once you're happy with your new way of eating and exercising – stick with it! This will get you the best possible results and mean you can maintain your body more easily. Enjoy your body and make sure your healthy lifestyle becomes a lifetime habit. If you choose to follow my six-week nutrition and exercise plan (pages 78–107 and pages 225–41), don't then go back to your old ways as soon as it's over. Those six weeks will prove to you what a healthy lifestyle can do for your body. Don't then go and throw it all away and binge for a week. Let the six-week plan be the beginning of a new chapter in your life. The way you feel about yourself will never be better and something that once was a burden will be easy to maintain FOR EVER!

 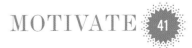

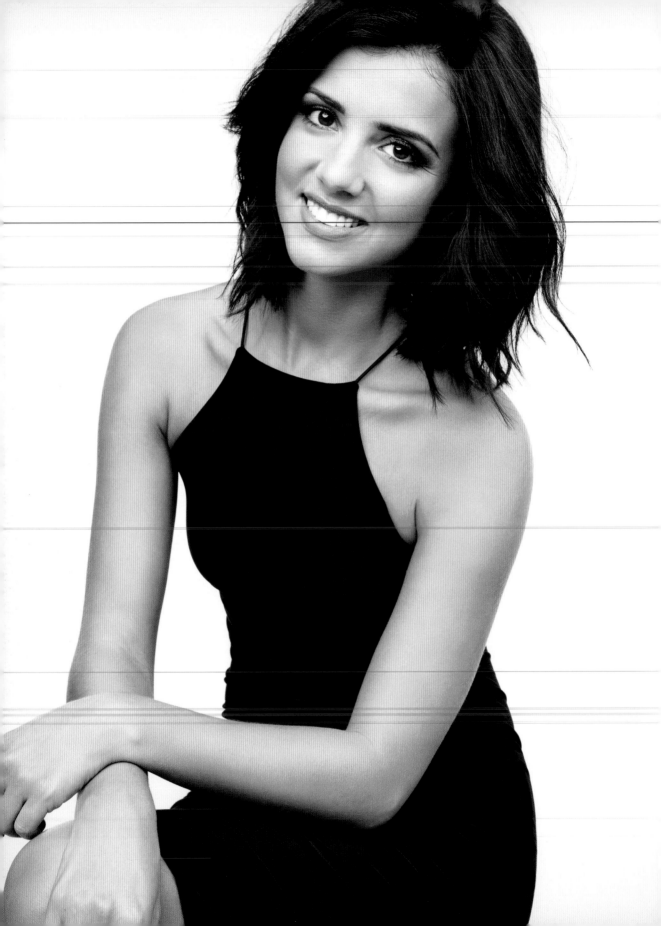

3
NOURISH

BAN THE WORD 'DIET' AND MAKE A LIFELONG CHANGE

For me, leading a healthy lifestyle is key to a happy life. It's like the most important insurance policy I could ever have. We don't need doctors or health experts to tell us the benefits of healthy living: it's widely known that the lifestyle choices you make on a daily basis can determine whether you are healthy or sick, gain weight or lose weight, feel happy or unhappy – your actions dictate your outcomes.

I've seen friends go through the experience of seeing someone that they care about having a health scare, and an experience like that changes your mentality. Your body is a fine-tuned machine and it can go wrong at any time – a bit like a car – but you can service it and make sure it's as fit as it possibly can be to try and avoid some of the more common problems.

For example, heart disease doesn't very often show itself until you are a lot older but it's what you do as a younger person that often dictates what happens to your body later in life. There are certain things that you can address and which will stop the damage being done to your cardiovascular system. This is something that I have really taken on board and I try and incorporate different foods in my diet to be able to fight diseases like this later in life. For so many illnesses, a healthy lifestyle is about prevention but really it's never too late to start. The human body is an amazing thing and it's never too late to help it naturally start to heal.

Raw juices daily are a great way to kick-start your immune system. My favourite is Lean and Green – try it and let me know what you think!

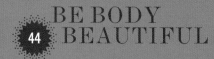

LEAN & GREEN JUICE

2 green apples
⅓ of a large cucumber
2 celery sticks
2 handfuls of curly kale
6 sprigs of fresh mint
   or parsley
1 lemon or lime

This juice takes a little while to prepare, so why not do it the night before? You can juice a load, then freeze the drinks and take one portion out of the freezer each night so it's defrosted by the morning.

• • ➔ •• • •• ➔ ••

Put all the ingredients through a juicer, then drink.

TIP
Juices can keep in the fridge air-sealed for no longer than 24 hours before they really lose their nutritional value. Adding lemon or lime preserves them better.

• • ➔ •• • •• ➔ ••

In the same way that heart disease can be combatted early by healthy eating and drinking options, so can a load of other chronic conditions. I can't emphasize enough how much your body is impacted by lifestyle and diet. Alzheimer's, arthritis, certain cancers, chronic fatigue syndrome, dementia, depression, diabetes, eczema and fibromyalgia are just a few conditions that can be really helped by what you eat and the respect you show your body. I know there's always exceptions to the rules and we all know someone who is really old and has never exercised a day in their life, cooked every vegetable to within an inch of its life, then coated it in table salt, smoked ten packets a day AND is rarely ever ill. But that's the exception to the rule. They probably just have good genes and a seriously efficient liver!

 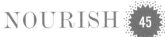

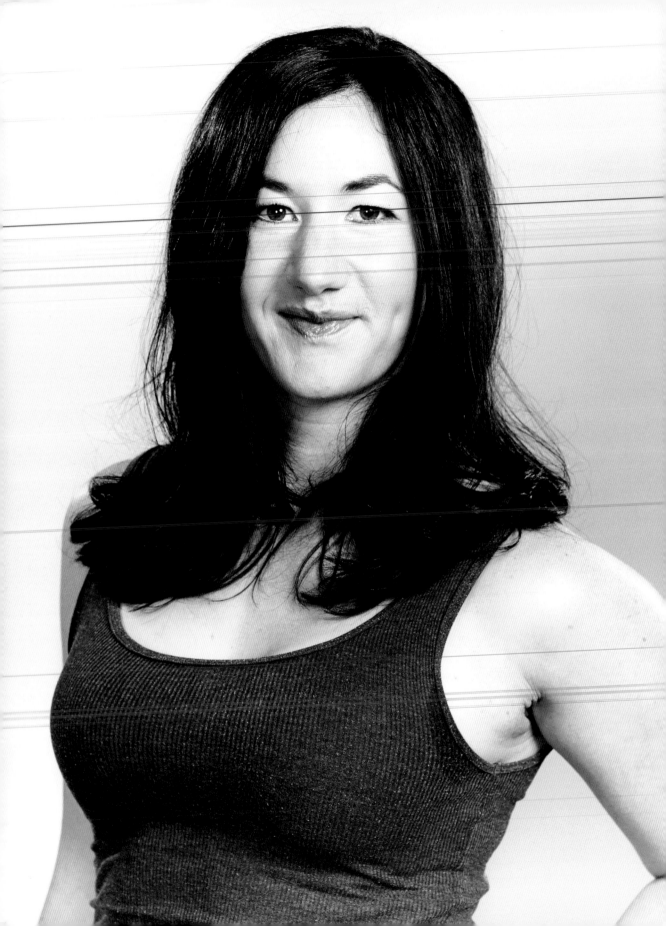

I met Emma Whitnall, a nutritional coach, when she joined my website team to create our online nutrition programmes. Straight away I organized a private appointment to see what I needed to be doing to make my own diet better. I didn't know a huge amount about nutrition. I knew what healthy food was but I never truly understood my body and how it worked. What surprised me most was that, although with her programmes I was effectively dieting, I could still eat so much, just of the right things. Packaging is often very misleading and you can get caught up in calories and fats, etc. It's the hidden things that you need to be worried about, but more of that later. Emma is amazing and has taught me so much. She has completely re-educated me when it comes to nutrition. One of the key things she says to me is, 'Stack the deck in your favour,' – meaning do as MUCH as you can, as OFTEN as you can to give your body the BEST POSSIBLE CHANCE of being healthy. Health is a massive priority for me now and always will be. With good health come great things!

I want to introduce you to Emma. What she doesn't know about nutrition isn't worth knowing. In this chapter, alongside Emma, I want to outline the ways you can change your life, like I did.

Emma can tell you a bit about me and what I was like when she first met me. She knows me better than most these days and is so motivational that I know once you've read this you'll want to join the club!

'STACK THE DECK IN YOUR
FAVOUR – DO AS MUCH
AS YOU CAN, AS OFTEN AS YOU CAN
TO GIVE YOUR BODY THE
BEST POSSIBLE CHANCE
OF BEING HEALTHY.'

 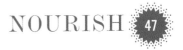

Lucy is one of the most determined people that I have ever met and for her exercise is key to her being happy. She loves it and it is her addiction on a day-to-day basis. My goal was to help Lucy maximize her training because nutrition contributes to 80% of results. We have a saying at Results with Lucy: 'Eat Clean, Train, Repeat' in that order.

At our first meeting, I remember Lucy being very smiley, warm and friendly and she was totally honest about everything. As part of my job I collate a lot of personal details from my clients, including a detailed description of bowel movements! And as our assessment went on, it transpired that digestion was in fact one of the issues Lucy needed help with. Following an in-depth body fat and lifestyle analysis, which included caliper testing to pinch body fat and a series of questionnaires on health history, diet history and general lifestyle, it was clear that, although she was in great shape, stress was another factor affecting her body and health, as were some obvious nutritional imbalances. Lucy's training sessions with Cecilia, her personal trainer, had already done wonders to improve her energy levels, but she

definitely needed a boost of B vitamins, to help manage stress, and a herbal cleanse, including liquid chlorophyll, to support digestion and clear away stored toxicity. I use a herbal cleanse supplement. Basically, it's a combination of detoxifying herbs, including yellow dock root, fenugreek, cranberry and many others, taken three times per day for ten days alongside drinking liquid chlorophyll in water. I developed my own detoxifying mixture, Mecktone, which essentially is a detoxifying health-food supplement. I take it daily because it's hard to get every nutrient your body needs. Mecktone is packed full of thirty healthy ingredients like cayenne pepper and aloe vera. It cleanses the skin and boosts metabolism: I love it.

One of the other main issues Lucy wanted help in addressing was water retention, including bloating around her belly, causing her (and I quote) 'to look six months pregnant'. Also, she would get physically sick with nerves, causing her to vomit, and this would happen at least once a week before I met her. There is a really strong connection between stress and digestion – we are all familiar with the sensation of nervous butterflies in our tummy – well for Lucy this connection

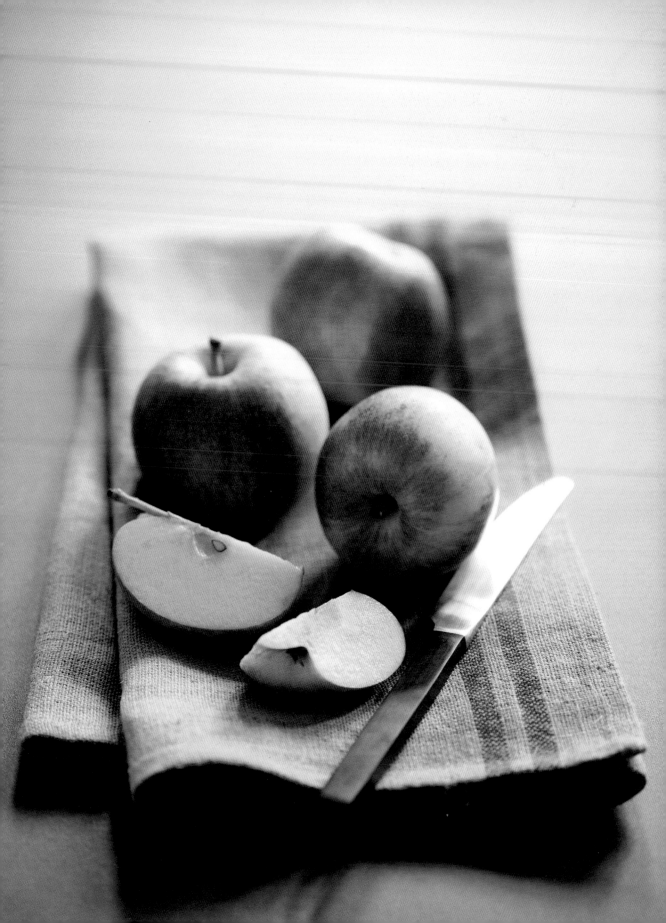

was intensified, I think, because of the pressure she was under being in the spotlight. Water retention and stomach bloating is a major issue for a lot of women and although hormones and food intolerances can play a role, I knew the herbal cleanse would really help her.

I recommended Lucy follow a nutrition plan that would first and foremost boost her health and as a fabulous side effect help to reduce cellulite and toxic body fat. This plan consisted of a lot of plant-based foods (loads of vegetables, raw juices, salads and super smoothies), with some animal proteins such as eggs, fish, chicken and occasional red meat, lots of healthy fats such as avocado, olive oil, coconut oil and oily fish, and gluten-free grains (quinoa, buckwheat and brown rice mainly). This plan of food and supplementation seemed to do the trick for months, with Lucy not having a single vomiting episode, until one day, a week before the pilot of *Tumble*, I received a text from Lucy, saying that she was nervous about the show and that her symptoms had returned – so I had to think of something that would reduce the nausea in time for the show (when in doubt turn to Mother Nature, and

sure enough she came through for Lucy!). The next day I met Lucy with a bag of fresh organic turmeric root and got her to juice about 15cm of turmeric with 5cm of ginger and a whole load of carrots and cucumber. You measure in centimetres because raw turmeric and ginger root are solid and long so you measure and cut off the correct amount. The juice had the desired effect and it stopped her stomach from churning and her feeling sick.

If you're feeling anxious, why not try this juice yourself? It's easy.

STOMACH-CALMING JUICE

4 carrots
¼ of a medium cucumber
2 green apples
15cm turmeric root
5cm ginger

SERVES 1
3-4 MINS TO MAKE

Put all the ingredients through a juicer and serve.

I know many people questioned Lucy's eating habits, I think because they were unable to comprehend that such an amazing figure can belong to someone who doesn't 'diet' or 'calorie count' but I want to set the record straight. Lucy loves her food and what works in her favour is that she doesn't calorie count or diet, because she keeps her body fuelled and constantly in 'fat-burning mode' with high-nutrient foods and, of course, does metabolic exercise, which includes squats, lunges, press-ups and burpees.

Lucy eats plenty of healthy nutritious fats like omega-3, found in salmon, eggs, flaxseeds and chia seeds, as well as the natural fats in avocado, nuts, seeds and coconut, which contribute to her flawless skin, and she gets numerous vitamins and minerals through raw vegetable juices. Lucy chooses to eat what I like to call 'Beauty Foods' which work for any 'body' wanting to maximize their physique and flaunt their beauty features. It doesn't matter your size or shape, eating for beauty works for everyone. If you want to flaunt your most appealing features then, like Lucy, you've got to get the nutrients in.

'IT DOESN'T MATTER, YOUR SIZE OR SHAPE, EATING FOR BEAUTY WORKS FOR EVERYONE.'

YOU CAN'T OUT-TRAIN A BAD DIET!

I thought my diet was relatively good until I met Emma but it was ridiculously bad and I needed an overhaul. You really can't out-train a bad diet. You need to stop it in its tracks and make a very definite change. The biggest thing to learn is that exercise and nutrition go hand in hand. One doesn't work efficiently without the other.

With Emma's help I will take you through the ways to make an instant change to your life as well as get rid of some of the myths about dieting.

Cellulite

Cellulite was my one major appearance bugbear and getting rid of it is something that I was successful in achieving. Loads of women suffer from cellulite and it's miserable. Plus, once you've got it, it's really hard to lose. Exercise played a major role in me getting rid of my cellulite and Cecilia's programmes were amazing, but to make sure cellulite goes away and stays away I needed to introduce anti-cellulite foods.

Emma says: 'Any foods that are high in antioxidants and at the same time detoxifying are perfect for reducing the appearance of cellulite. Foods such as green and white teas, berries, raw cocoa, chlorophyll taken in water – this is a liquid, you add about 1 teaspoon to around 600ml (1 pint) of water or a few drops in your drinking water throughout the day – spirulina and wheatgrass all help to reduce the free-radical damage and inflammation that cause cellulite to appear, as well as removing the toxins that get stored in areas of cellulite. Once these foods have done their job, exercise is critical for increasing blood flow and lymphatic drainage. You get the idea: one without the other is a half job, and so both exercise and nutrition are a winning combination for results.'

'A DAILY INTAKE OF DETOXIFYING
FOODS IS KEY
TO HEALTHY SUSTAINABLE
WEIGHT LOSS.'

MAKING THE CHANGE SOUNDS HARDER THAN IT IS

At first it seems really hard to incorporate all these different things into your life. It seems weird to start drinking teas that you've never heard of before or eating random foods, but once you start to see the results then I think that spurs you on – I know it did with me. So often people give up before they even start to make healthier lifestyle changes because they think it's too much effort or they find it totally overwhelming. Make things simple and easy to follow so that you don't feel bogged down by it all. Make the changes part of your life as opposed to extra things to do and that way they will work around you rather than the other way around.

Emma says: 'Aside from the undeniably desirable result of having less cellulite there are MANY other benefits of healthy eating and healthy living, such as: increased energy; better brain function and productivity at work; better skin, hair and nails; to easily reduce body weight; to recover from stress and injury more efficiently; to have healthier children; to conceive and carry more easily in pregnancy; and, of course, the big one, to reduce your chances of living your later years in and out of hospital, relying on a cocktail of medications.'

One of the biggest myths I had believed was that I would have to start missing out on the good things in life. How many times have I heard people say that 'life is for living: you're only here once so don't deprive yourself'? Too many times. If you don't eat healthily, life won't be there to live. However, it's important not to make healthy living anti-social and there's no need for it to be.

Emma says: 'Many of my clients have a fear of missing out while living healthily, which is far from the truth. To me an important part of healthy living is being sociable and enjoying life. No one benefits from feeling isolated because of his or her lifestyle choices. Therefore

BE BODY BEAUTIFUL

LUCY AND EMMA'S TOP TIPS FOR
MAKING A HEALTHY LIFE CHANGE

1 Find your motivation (your 'Why').

2 Exercise doing what you love. If you hate running then don't run! Find something else.

3 Find healthy foods you enjoy. You have plenty to choose from in the recipes in this book (pages 151–223).

4 Make ONE change at a time and master it. It might be that you aim to drink more water or swap your pasta for quinoa or add in an extra green vegetable every day. Choose things that are simple, doable and effective.

5 Make time. We all have the same 24 hours in a day – it's your choice what you do in those hours.

6 Don't use family as an excuse. Far too many people (women in particular) hide behind their family as an excuse to stay unhealthy and unhappy with their bodies.

7 Work in success. Always set a goal that is slightly out of reach but still attainable. Nothing will make you want to give up faster than perceived failure.

8 Seek help. Everyone needs a coach or someone to help them – if you can, get one. You are not expected to be superwoman and know it all!

 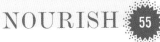

it's about getting the balance right, it's the 80/20 rule. 80% of the time do as MUCH as you can, as OFTEN as you can to give your body the BEST POSSIBLE CHANCE of being healthy, and then 20% of the time eat, drink and do as you please! Have a night out with the girls, order a dessert in a restaurant, order the naan AND the rice. Just don't do it every other night. It's not the one cheat or treat that will cause ill health or add on the pounds; it's when they become a part of your '80' that they start to be detrimental. What I do find time and again is that the longer people live a healthy lifestyle, the better they feel, the better they look and their natural desires start to move away from wanting the foods that are no good for them. Soon one or two glasses of wine becomes satisfying as opposed to the whole bottle.'

I made the change because I wanted to. My life experiences and being on *TOWIE* all affected me and they made me want to actively make a change to the way I felt and to the way I looked. I wanted to take control of my body rather than it taking control over me. I think most people need that epiphany, if you like, to make them see the light! To make them really want something badly enough that they are willing to make some quite big changes in the first instance.

Emma says: 'I believe in order to be successful in change you must find the most meaningful reason to do so. I call this your "Why" – which might be to remain on this earth long enough to see your children and grandchildren grow up, or to increase your energy and fitness levels to make you the BEST candidate for the job promotion you've been after or it might simply be to gain the satisfaction of looking drop-dead gorgeous every time you see your ex. Whatever your reason, it has to be good enough to keep you from wavering, from wobbling and giving up at the first hurdle because, trust me, there will be more than one hurdle. If in the past you have attempted to lose weight or run a marathon and you have given up too easily, either the plan wasn't right or your reason for starting in the first place wasn't meaningful enough! I mean this sincerely when I say if you really struggle to find something worthy of a healthier lifestyle, then try starting with YOU! You are the most valid reason I can think of, 100%.'

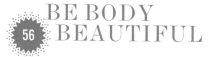

A lot of people would never even think of a nutrition or exercise coach because they think it's expensive and I do get that everyone has a different budget but it's about priorities. How many dresses have you bought this month? How many times have you had your nails done? Put health advice into perspective. How important is being healthy to you? Emma has made a huge difference to my quality of life. Not only physically changing my body but giving me a totally different mental outlook. I work hard and I make sure I put enough money aside for quality organic produce and organic skin products. I'd rather go without a few Starbucks coffees than go without these things. I see it as an investment in my health and hopefully, when the time comes, my children's health too.

Emma says: 'If you don't look after your body, where else are you going to live? Just think about this whenever you feel like buying a cheaper product instead of taking care of the things that will ultimately take care of you.'

We live in a 'now' society. Everything is accessible and immediate and, in the same way, when we start to make changes to our diet and exercise regimes we want to see results pretty much immediately. Mix exercise and changing your diet and I think the results ARE pretty much immediate. I know that when I eat a diet high in nutrient-dense foods, when I exercise regularly and when I manage my stress I immediately have greater energy, a more robust immune system, a flatter belly and greater confidence in my physical and mental fitness, knowing that I can more easily deal with any scenario that life throws my way.

When you lead a healthy lifestyle something amazing happens, an empowering change takes place within you. When you start to see changes in your body, when niggles, aches, pains and allergies start to subside and you no longer get uncontrollable cravings, you feel incredible knowing that you and you alone made that happen… Nothing beats that feeling.

 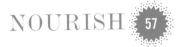

WHAT ARE THE BEST FOODS TO EAT?

There is so much information out there and a lot of it is conflicting. If you don't know a lot about food then it's really tricky. All the crap on the packaging doesn't seem to simplify what we all want to know. Which foods really are the healthy ones? Which foods will not only promote weight loss and toning but also enhance beauty features like hair, skin and nails?

I was always confused until Emma basically educated me on it all. I had very specific goals – get healthy, gain lean muscle, drop body fat, get a 'six-pack' and bust the cellulite. But, there are unshakable TRUTHS, or principles, that must be applied. Emma says: 'I taught Lucy my three health and fat-loss truths early on in our coaching and now I have developed numerous programs for Results with Lucy founded upon these same ideas. You can use these truths like a checklist to qualify your future food choices.'

Truth 1:
Count Nutrients NOT Calories

If you want to create an optimum environment for your body to lose body fat, increase lean tissue or shed abdominal fat, you need to up the nutrients and NOT reduce the calories. Calorie restriction stresses the body, disturbing your metabolism and restricting the very nutrients that work to burn body fat and build lean tissue. Food provides your cells with information, which on a daily basis can signal you to be healthy, or not, and in turn to lose weight, or not. Foods that are high in natural nutrition tend also to be low in calories anyway; good to know if, as a die-hard dieter or former calorie-counter, this concept takes you a while to get used to.

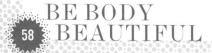

Truth 2:
Don't Diet – Detoxify

One of the messages I am very passionate about getting across to women in particular is that diets don't work. It makes intuitive sense that diets are the WRONG approach, but sometimes desperation leads us to do things we know are not good for us and that is why I ALWAYS get my clients to DETOXIFY as opposed to dieting. Lucy is no exception to this. A daily intake of detoxifying foods is key for healthy sustainable fat loss. Detox also clears out toxins that prevent nutrients getting into cells (preventing lean muscle gain and fat loss), which is why so many of my clients achieve incredible results when on a herbal detox and taking liquid chlorophyll.

A herbal detox basically means an elimination of sugar, alcohol, caffeine, gluten, cow dairy and processed foods for a minimum of ten days, whilst eating high-nutrient foods such as those in Eat Mostly category (pages 61–2) – proteins, vegetables, fruits, eggs, seeds, nuts and lots of raw juices and green smoothies containing kale, spinach, berries, etc – at the same time taking the healthy starter pack herbal cleanse I mentioned earlier.

Truth 3:
Balance Your Hormones – Especially Insulin

Many women are afraid of eating fat for fear it will make them exactly that. But the truth is that sugar, high-fructose corn syrup and highly refined carbohydrates, such as those in breads, pasta, sweets, cakes, biscuits and processed foods, are the main culprits in weight gain. When I get clients to increase their healthy fat intake, while decreasing their refined-sugar intake they cannot believe the changes in their bodies. Very quickly they become leaner, stronger and more energized. Insulin is the hormone that is produced in response to sugar (and all carbs) and although without it we would ultimately die, in excess it becomes a powerful fat-storing hormone.

Emma has got me to think properly about my food and make informed choices. So now, when I go shopping, I try to make it easy for myself and I ask myself a few basic questions while I'm deciding what to buy. I appreciate there isn't always the time to think and you just need to chuck it in the trolley and go but, if you can, try and ask yourself:

ARE YOUR FOODS . . .

1 Nourishing – High in vitamins, minerals, antioxidants, fats, fibre and protein?

2 Detoxifying – Natural, clean foods, high in antioxidants, vitamins, minerals, amino acids and free from processing, chemicals, additives, flavour enhancers and artificial sweeteners?

3 Balancing (blood sugar) – High in fibre and/or protein, low-glycemic load, unrefined whole foods?

•·◆·•◦·•◦·◆·•◦

Emma says: 'Any food that ticks all three of the above criteria goes into my Eat Mostly category. Remember the 80/20 Rule that I have? This is how it works and here's how to apply it. Get 80% of your weekly food from the Eat Mostly and Eat Moderately lists and, if you choose to, 20% from the Eat Occasionally and Eat Rarely lists.'

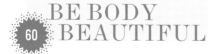

Eat Mostly

Low-starch/High-fibre Vegetables

These should make up the foundation of everybody's daily diet as they provide the highest doses of vitamins, minerals and antioxidants. They aid in digestion and keeping your bowels regular, as well as supporting many weight-loss processes in the body.

High-fibre vegetables include artichokes, asparagus, bamboo shoots, sprouts, pak choi, broccoli, cabbage, carrots, cauliflower, celery, courgettes, chives and kale.

Animal and Plant Proteins

Protein, be it from animal or plant sources, is made up of amino acids, which are required to repair and rebuild skin, hair and muscle tissue and help to keep hormones balanced. Protein is very filling and does not spike blood-sugar levels, making it a great fat-burning and muscle-toning companion. Many of my female clients are initially a bit scared of protein, having the misconception that if they eat protein with every meal or add a protein supplement to their smoothies suddenly they'll start to bulk up, but this simply is not true. It takes a very specific type of training and more protein than you could easily consume in any given day to start getting 'bulking effects' from eating protein. Protein includes chicken, turkey, duck, fish, seafood and free-range eggs (animal sources); quinoa, spirulina, legumes such as kidney, pinto and black beans, green peas, soya beans, lentils, chickpeas and all nuts (vegetable sources).

Low–medium Glycemic Load Foods and Highly Antioxidant Fruits

Glycemic load (GL) basically determines how much a food will raise blood-sugar levels (and in turn insulin). Fruits are some of the most nutrient-dense foods on the planet. Like the fibrous vegetables listed above, they contain powerful antioxidants that are cleansing, anti-ageing and fat-burning. Fruits get a bad reputation because they contain sugar, but so long as that sugar is consumed with the fibre of the fruit, its GL remains low–medium. All fruit is good, and fresh is best: apples, apricots, avocados, bananas, all berries, cherries, fresh figs, dried goji berries, grapes, grapefruit, kiwi fruit, mandarins, mango, melon, nectarines, oranges, passion fruit, peaches, pears, pineapple, tangerines and tomatoes.

Flash-frozen fruit retains nearly all of the nutrients and in some cases such as blueberries can actually increase the antioxidant and nutritional content.

Low–medium Glycemic Load Starchy Vegetables and Gluten-free Grains

Most starchy vegetables, though high in carbs, have a low–medium glycemic load. The lower the GL the better for weight loss.

Good starchy vegetables include: carrots, celeriac, parsnips, pumpkin, squash, sweet potatoes, swede, turnips and yams. Gluten-free grains are: amaranth, buckwheat, brown rice, millet and quinoa.

Healthy Fats, Seeds and Nuts

Good fats are in fact fat-burning and a deficiency in any essential fats can slow metabolism, slow weight loss and lead to chronic diseases such as heart disease and diabetes.

Good fats include: all nuts, all seeds (especially ground flaxseeds and chia seeds), coconut and its oil, olives and olive oil, avocados and their oil, oily fish and organic butter.

Cleansing Drinks

You can't move nutrients around the body to get rid of toxins without cleansing drinks. Aim for 2–3 litres of water per day. Staying hydrated is one of the most frequently overlooked 'musts' for weight loss and fat loss.

Try filtered water, liquid chlorophyll, lemon and hot water, fresh raw vegetable and fruit juices, fruit-infused filtered water and herbal teas – especially green and white teas.

Eat Moderately

The following foods don't necessarily fit with all three 'truths', but still contain certain nutritional benefits including fibre, low GL, vitamins, minerals and proteins:

★ Wheat-free grains (barley, corn, oats, spelt, rye)
★ Red meat (lamb, venison, beef)
★ Organic milk (if lactose tolerant)
★ Plain yogurt (if lactose tolerant)
★ Goat's cheese
★ Feta cheese
★ Tea and coffee
★ Dark chocolate (70%+ cocoa solids)

Eat Occasionally

The following foods are best only consumed occasionally; they are either too processed, too toxic or too high on the GL scale to fit into the 80% eating regime.

★ White potatoes
★ Basmati or jasmine rice
★ Wheat (conventional bread, pasta, cereals, bakery items, pastries, biscuits)

BE BODY BEAUTIFUL

★ Alcohol
★ Real ice cream and other dairy products, such as sour cream, cream cheese, cottage cheese, fruit yogurts (except those with the artificial sweetener aspartame)

Eat Rarely or Never

The following are highly processed, toxic to the body and are linked not only to weight gain, but disease as well:
★ Refined sugar (as found in processed milk chocolate, sweets and junk foods)
★ Fructose (on its own) and high-fructose corn syrup
★ Hydrogenated fats (as in margarine)
★ Factory-made frozen desserts ('pretend' ice cream)
★ Artificial sweeteners, especially aspartame (found abundantly in diet sodas and yogurts, low-fat/low-calorie products, chewing gum and mint sweets)
★ MSG – a flavour enhancer that is mostly found in junk foods such as Pringles, Doritos and Chinese foods (including sauces and stock powders)

A Note on Organic Food

By now you will have some idea of the importance of a 'clean system' for health and weight loss. Chemical sprays that bombard our crops and genetically modified foods add to our daily toxic burden so part of keeping the body clean (remember Emma's second 'truth') is to opt as often as possible for organic produce.

In July 2014, a study conducted at Newcastle University was published in the *British Journal of Nutrition* that proved organic fruits, vegetables and cereals, and foods made from them, to be up to 60% more nutritious than conventionally grown produce, meaning the added nutrition and the lack of toxins makes it worth the small additional investment.

Those principles Emma gave me are what I pretty much live by and they have made me who I am today. Gone are the days of me skipping breakfast, having a sandwich for lunch and pasta for tea. What I was doing doesn't sound bad but if you look at the nutrition I was getting there was barely any at all, just a whole lot of nutrient-devoid refined carbohydrates. It's no wonder I had energy and digestive issues!

Does anyone else suffer from chocolate cravings? I used to get them so badly at night. And I've come to know that is a classic sign that your body is not getting enough protein or vitamins and minerals.

I soon put a stop to my cravings by introducing a protein-rich breakfast, which is probably one of my favourite meals (especially salmon scrambled eggs and avocado on German rye bread).

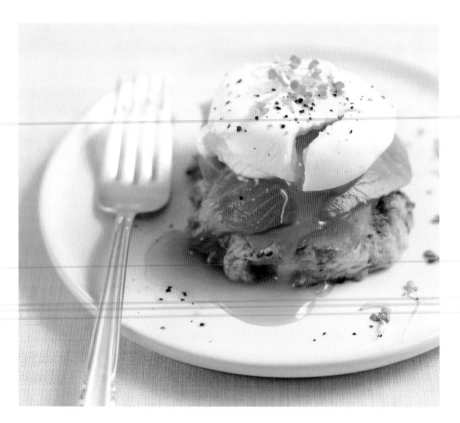

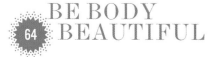

BE BODY
BEAUTIFUL

Lunches became salads with protein, and evening meals a mix of protein with vegetables and a healthy carb option, such as quinoa or a baked sweet potato. If I did get a craving, I swapped the sugary milk chocolate I had eaten before in the evenings for an organic dark variety (70%+ cocoa solids), which has nearly half the amount of sugar in it as common milk chocolate brands.

Chocolate cravings are a very real thing for many women, especially around certain times of the month. We crave chocolate partly for the feel-good buzz that sugar gives us but mainly our bodies want the magnesium and iron contained in the cocoa itself. A great way to deal with pre-menstrual chocolate and sugar cravings is to feed your body more iron- and magnesium-rich foods throughout your cycle (not just in the lead up to your period). Green vegetables and green smoothies are particularly good! One of my absolute favourite 'craving-proof' snacks is the following raw chocolate mud shake.

RAW CHOCOLATE MUD SHAKE

flesh of ½ an avocado
1 banana
120ml almond milk
2 tsp raw organic liquid
honey or agave (a popular
natural sweetener)
2 tsp Green and Blacks
dark cocoa powder
1 tsp raw cocoa nibs
240ml filtered water

SERVES 1
2–3 MINS TO MAKE

A delicious and healthy way to beat chocolate cravings.

•• •◆ •• •◆ ••

Combine all the ingredients in a high-speed blender, adding more water if the consistency is too thick.

 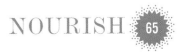

Sugar: The Truth

Emma has taught me a lot and one of things is that sugar is not your friend. Seriously, not only can it very easily derail your weight-loss attempts because of its affect on insulin (which can play a role in weight gain), but there are other health-related issues when it comes to table sugar (sucrose). It's a man-made, highly refined, highly addictive substance. In many people sugar creates an addictive response, which can lead to all sorts of problems – weight gain being just one of them.

Emma says: 'Fructose is another form of sugar that comes naturally from fruits and vegetables. In amounts consumed through a diet of the Eat Mostly category foods (see pages 61–2), the body can metabolize and process fructose no problem at all. But refined fructose, which is when the sugar is extracted from fruit (without the fibre, enzymes and antioxidants that should be consumed with it), has caused HUGE health problems in terms of obesity, diabetes and heart disease over the past 20–30 years. Excessive amounts of fructose coming into the body these days through sugary and syrupy drinks, such as fizzy drinks, fruit juices, flavoured coffees and frappuccinos, are causing many people to get chronic liver diseases such as cirrhosis – historically only associated with excess alcohol consumption. Too much sugar (fructose in particular) is as damaging to the liver as excess alcohol.

Before I understood the damaging effects of sugar, I would always drink sugary cocktails, but now when I go on a night out with the girls (as part of my 80/20 programme), I opt for a red wine or a vodka and soda, both of which have far less sugar.

Why Go Wheat and Gluten Free?

More and more people are finding that gluten is a key contributor to their niggles and ailments; even those that aren't necessarily 'allergic' to gluten (celiac) may still have an intolerance which can cause bloating, excess gas and intestinal pain and swelling. If you

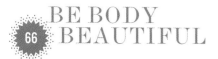

aren't gluten intolerant or allergic, then Emma recommends you opt for eating moderate amounts of porridge oats or German rye bread as a replacement for processed breakfast cereals and toast. I swap cereals and toast for these all of the time and I rarely feel bloated.

Emma says: 'Gluten is sticky by nature (hence it's name *glu*-ten) and if it doesn't cause an inflammatory immune response in the body, it may still bind to the digestive wall, slowing digestion and interfering with nutrient absorption. Gluten is a protein found in many grains, including wheat. This tends to be the more 'offensive' gluten, but the gluten in barley, spelt and rye can also cause people issues.'

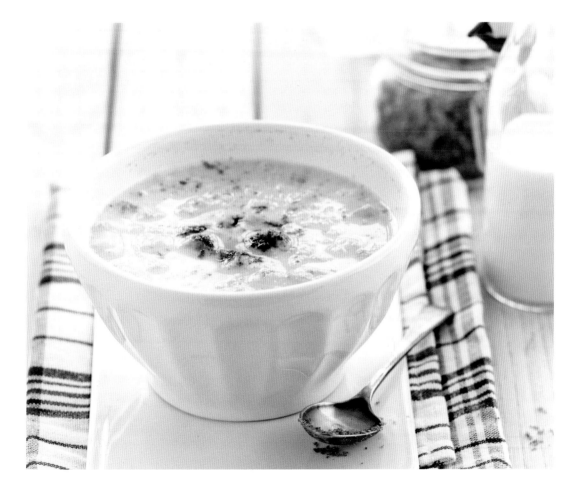

 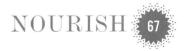

Beauty Foods

They say beauty is in the eye of the beholder, but for me it's also in the food that you eat! From weight loss all the way through to having radiant skin, glossy hair and strong healthy nails, undoubtedly beauty foods are the way forwards! They also have the added bonus of being good for the waistline and good for digestion, plus they are anti-ageing, not only for your skin, but for your insides too!

I eat a load of essential fats which are one of the best beauty foods you can eat because they give your skin cells a full and smooth appearance, as well as helping to stop dry, scaly skin and dry, damaged hair. Omega-3 is an essential fat; mono- and polyunsaturated fats, such as those found in olives, avocados, seeds and nuts, are also essential fats.

I'm currently totally obsessed with beauty minerals, such as sulphur, zinc, manganese, silicon and iron; and Emma is creating meals with foods high in the following to ensure my skin remains as young as it can for as long as it can:

★ **Sulphur** – needed for glossy hair and skin complexion and elasticity. Found in cabbage, kale, rocket, garlic, broccoli and Brussels sprouts!

★ **Zinc** – needed for skin health but also to help balance hormones. Found in seeds, nuts, coconut, spinach, spirulina (a blue–green algae from the sea that is incredibly high in antioxidants, and vitamins and minerals such as calcium, magnesium and B vitamins to name a few) and other seaweeds.

★ **Silicon** – needed for bone mineral density, prevention of gum disease, shiny and strong hair, strong nails and a toned complexion. Found in rosemary, horsetail (a herb), alfalfa (a legume belonging to the pea family which is typically added to salads as alfalfa sprouts), romaine lettuce, spinach, burdock root, radishes, cucumber, capsicums (sweet and chilli peppers), tomatoes and oats.

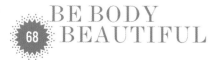

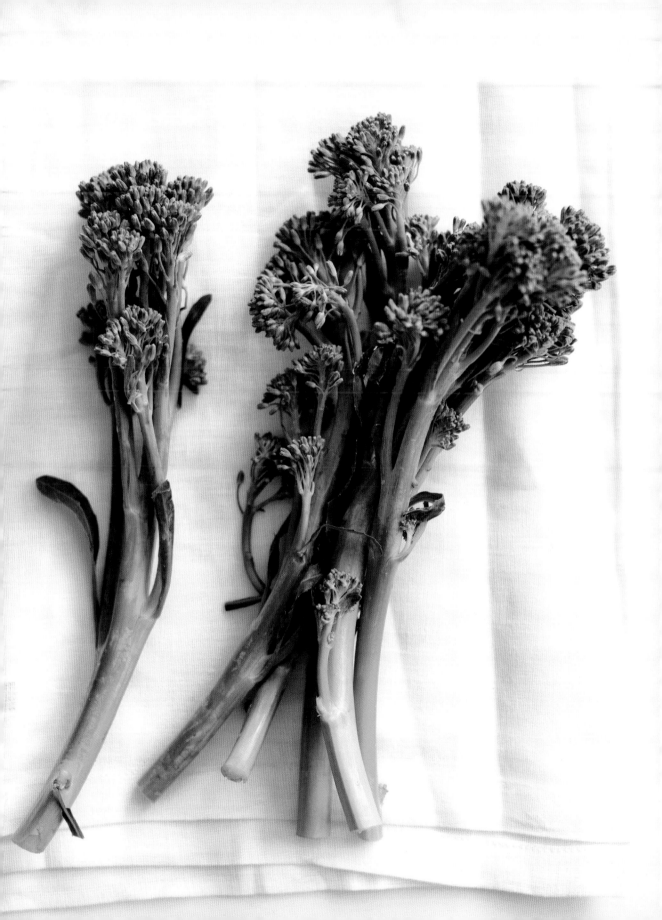

★ **Manganese** – needed to produce connective tissue for a toned complexion. Found in cloves, cocoa beans, hemp seeds, nuts, spinach, watercress, kale, raisins, prunes and sweet potatoes.

★ **Iron** – helps to carry oxygen to all cells (because dead cells = premature ageing and dull, lifeless and limp beauty features). Hair thinning and breaking can also be a sign of iron deficiency. Found in meat, beans and nuts.

You will notice that beauty nutrients are found mostly in plant-based foods and, as well as being great for your beauty features, they are also the best foods to eat for health and weight loss...

REMEMBER: The best nutrition programme should make you HEALTHY on the inside, SEXY on the outside and HAPPY everywhere in the middle. Don't ever forget that!

Here's mine and Emma's 'Happy, Sexy, Healthy Programme'. Stick to it and lose up to 10 pounds of body fat, or a dress size, and reduce the appearance of cellulite in just six weeks.

This two-step programme uses the F.E.M. (FOOD, EXERCISE, MASSAGE) formula. Over the course of the next six weeks this programme will help you:

★ Reduce the appearance of cellulite
★ Reduce overall body fat
★ Improve skin health and tone current areas of cellulite

Before I set out our two-step plan I want to try and explain what cellulite is because I think cellulite is one of those things that all women at some point in their life struggle with. I have never been especially overweight yet I have still suffered from it. Why do we have it? And how the hell do we get rid of it?

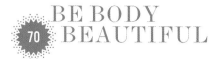

Emma says: 'The medical term for cellulite is dermo-panniculosis deformans, which basically means a tethering of the deep layers of the skin (elastin fibres in particular) to the underlying muscle. This essentially squeezes the fat cells that sit between the muscle and the skin on top, creating an uneven and dimpled appearance. In true cellulite cases, anatomical changes can actually be detected under a microscope. These physical changes have nothing to do with your body fat per se, but the elastic fibres of the skin which connect your muscle tissue and skin together. However, enlarged fat cells where you can detect more cellulite are usually full of toxins. (Our fat cells are the safest and most logical place for toxic storage in the body.) Therefore toxic build-up within the body is a sure contributor to the appearance of cellulite.

'Cellulite-affected areas, such as on the bottom and at the tops of the thighs, typically show the associated symptoms of low blood flow and poor circulation. It is unknown if these are part of the cause of cellulite, or part of its effects, but one thing we do know is that if circulation is poor, toxins will get stuck and collect in those areas, adding to the cellulite burden.'

I could never really understand how I'd suddenly got cellulite but a lot of it is down to your DNA. The good news is that with most genes they are only triggered by the environment in which they exist. The exact environmental trigger of cellulite remains unknown for sure, however is noticeably linked to:

★ Poor circulation
★ Lack of antioxidants in the diet
★ Toxic build up – smoking, alcohol, caffeine, sugar
★ Sluggish liver (some people have a lower tolerance for toxins)
★ Hormonal imbalance – particularly relating to stress and menstrual hormones
★ Poor food choices

•• ◆• •◆• •◆• •◆• ••

 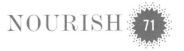

Processed foods, chemical-laden foods, high-sugar foods (but notice I didn't say fatty foods) all contribute to increased cellulite appearance. Stress alone can be enough to see changes in skin elasticity. When you are stressed, your hormones can change. We use up more antioxidants from our diet to battle the stress, leaving fewer antioxidants to take care of the health of our skin. Plus, very often we turn to more sugary toxic foods when stressed. There are a number of ways to combat the orange-peel skin of cellulite. Forget those topical procedures and creams – I don't think you will ever achieve the body you want sans cellulite unless you knuckle down, exercise and change your diet.

The food we choose to eat on a daily basis will ultimately determine the aesthetic outcomes we get. Emma says: 'Food carries important information by way of nutrients to our cells and, depending on the messages they carry, we get more fat-storage or fat-loss results. A high intake of antioxidants and detoxifying foods can dramatically offset the appearance of cellulite.'

I am exercise's number-one fan so for me this is a given but, of course, it goes without saying that exercise plays a major role in the elimination of cellulite. One of the well-known risk factors for cellulite, as outlined above, is poor circulation to the affected areas. Exercise increases blood flow and therefore good nutrients get delivered to the affected cells and toxic waste that the food and supplements are clearing out from the affected area can get carried away efficiently.

Brilliantly, massage is another fantastic circulation and detoxification stimulant. Apart from being a great excuse to get pampered, booking yourself a weekly lymphatic drainage massage is highly recommended to enhance the results you will get if you follow our programme. If it is not possible for you to book a regular massage, we highly recommend dry body brushing on a daily basis.

Here we go. We've explained each step so that you know exactly what you are trying to achieve and to give you a better understanding of how your body works. Lose 10 pounds and a dress size in six weeks. Go on, give it a go.

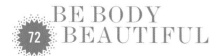

'THE FOOD WE CHOOSE TO **EAT** ON A DAILY BASIS **WILL** ULTIMATELY DETERMINE **THE OUTCOME WE GET.'**

THE TWO-STEP PROGRAMME

STEP 1:
'Clean and Clear' Weeks 1–3

No matter what physical goal you set out to achieve, there is one solid fact that remains true throughout and that is that a 'clean' body is a lean body! And … given the role that toxicity plays in cellulite, detoxification and clearing toxic residue from fat cells is an essential place to start.

The Oestrogen Relationship and Cellulite

Oestrogen is a DOMINANT hormone and very influential on fat storage. It is responsible partly for the distribution of fat around the hips and the thighs. Healthy oestrogen metabolism relies heavily on your intake of cruciferous vegetables (broccoli, cabbage, kale, etc.) and your liver health. Oestrogen metabolites, if not cleared properly by the liver, can get trapped in fatty tissue, therefore adding to the cellulite burden.

Pollution in our environment, alcohol, lack of antioxidant intake, stress and processed soya products are to name just a few factors that contribute to imbalances in oestrogen (in both men and women), but don't panic because step one of this programme is all about clearing out toxic hormonal by-products and rebalancing your system through cleansing and detoxifying foods!

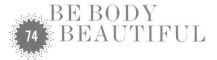

STEP 2:
'Nourish and Repair' Weeks 4–6

A contributing factor to the appearance of cellulite is the physical changes that take place in the muscle and skin cells. Keeping your muscles well nourished and toned (through the exercise component of your plan) is crucial for successful results.

Protein is required to repair and rebuild skin and muscle, and to help keep hormones balanced – especially insulin, which we know is a prominent fat-storage hormone. Hence, it's important to get enough protein power into your diet!

Recommended Plant Proteins for this Plan:
★ Legumes (all peas, beans and lentils)
★ Quinoa
★ Spirulina (powder or capsules) – a superfood since it contains all eight essential amino acids; something to consider taking to boost protein intake and help to alkalize the body
★ Naturally fermented/non-GM soya (tofu and tempeh)

Recommended Animal Proteins:
★ Eggs
★ Poultry
★ Fresh fish
★ Seafood

The Importance of Antioxidants in Cellulite Prevention and Elimination

Antioxidants are the anti-ageing, disease-fighting, skin- and cell-repairing nutrients contained within plant-based foods that fight off free-radical damage and prevent unwanted changes to our cells. They are Mother Nature's gifts to us for longevity and beauty!

 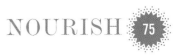

Basically antioxidants mop up free radicals, which damage our cells and tissues. Free radicals are generated by-products of normal metabolism, but the toxins we are exposed to like the sun and alcohol can also cause free-radical damage to our cells and cause premature cell death or mutation.

Antioxidants have many guises including:
- ★ **Vitamins and co-factors** – specifically vitamins A, C, E and Co Q10
- ★ **Hormones** – melatonin (sleep hormone)
- ★ **Minerals** – selenium, manganese, magnesium, zinc and iodine
- ★ **Phytonutrients** – beta carotene (found in carrots and oranges), lycopene (from tomatoes), flavonoids (in berries, nuts, green and white teas), phenolics (found in turmeric, cinnamon and oregano)
- ★ **Omega-3** – an essential fatty acid that signals to the body to switch ON your fat-burning enzymes and switch OFF your fat-storing enzymes (and also helps to maintain the integrity of your skin cells – keeping them looking healthy!)

We recommend taking an omega-3 supplement but make sure you are buying a quality product. From an ethical stance the omega-3 should come from sustainably sourced fish and use the oil from the whole fish's body, not just the liver. A good-quality brand will guarantee being free from mercury, radiation and pesticide residues and be pure and stable so that the capsules do not turn rancid easily.

'SWITCH ON YOUR
FAT-BURNING ENZYMES
AND SWITCH OFF YOUR
FAT-STORING ENZYMES!'

BE BODY
BEAUTIFUL

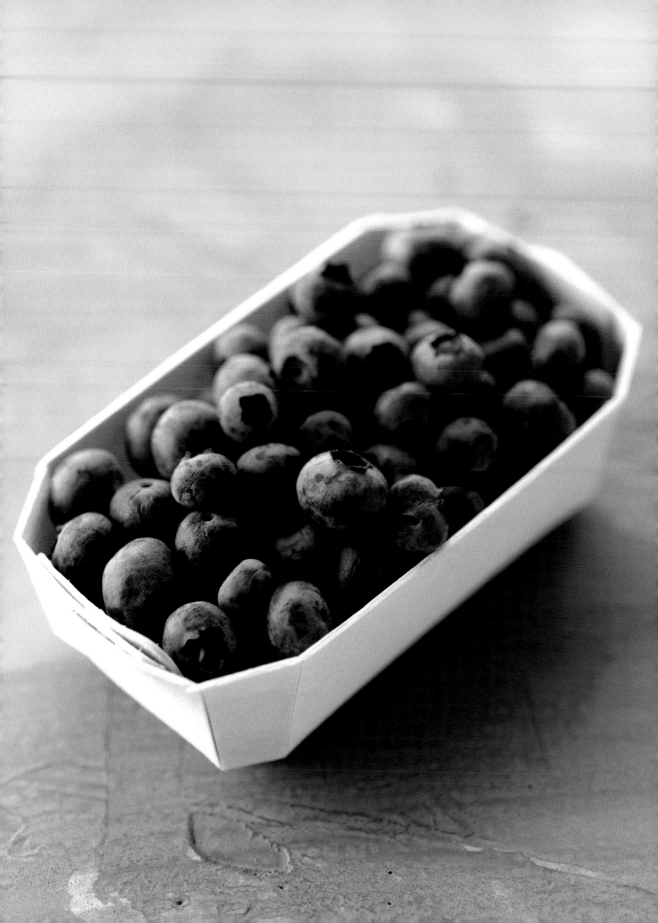

THE PLAN:
STEP 1 – CLEAN & CLEAR
(WEEKS 1–3)

Week 1: 'Cutting the C*@p'

It's time to clear out the sugars, toxic fats and artificial ingredients that may be going into your current daily diet.

Nutrition Tasks for 'Clean and Clear' Week 1 (days 1–7)

Here is a list of six no-no foods and ingredients you MUST eliminate this week.

NO-NOS	WHY ELIMINATE	REPLACE WITH	BUY FROM
Margarine and vegetable oil spreads.	Margarines and other vegetable oil spreads contain high levels of hydrogenated (man-made) fats, which the body cannot process. They are toxic and lead to weight gain!	Organic butter, avocado, raw nut butters (cashew, almond, hazelnut), extra virgin olive oil and coconut oil.	Supermarkets or health-food stores.
Aspartame Found in artificial sweeteners (such as Equal, Sweet'N Low and Splenda) and in all diet sodas, flavoured waters, low-sugar drinks and cordials, and most low-fat products (such as yogurts).	This artificial sweetener has proven to be toxic to the brain and nervous system in some individuals – simulating symptoms in line with those of multiple sclerosis. Aspartame has also been linked to weight gain.	Stevia, raw honey, agave nectar.	Supermarkets, Wholefoods or your local health-food store.

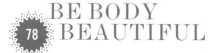

NO-NOS	WHY ELIMINATE	REPLACE WITH	BUY FROM
Sugar/sugary products Such as brown and white table sugar; sweets; puddings; milk chocolate; low-fat products; fruit yogurts; fruit juice (in cartons, cans and bottles); cordials and squash; Innocent smoothies and other bottled smoothies; cereal bars (which contain wheat anyway); dried fruits such as mango, pineapple, dried bananas; ready meals (which contain hydrogenated fats anyway); tinned fruit; hot chocolate N.B. This list is not exhaustive.	Table sugar (sucrose) is a man-made, highly refined, highly addictive substance, which health authorities are now viewing like a drug! Similar to the class-A drug cocaine (a white substance produced by the extensive refining and processing of the coca plant), sugar is also a highly refined and processed white substance that comes from a natural plant (sugar cane). In many people sugar creates an addictive response, which can lead to all sorts of problems – weight gain being one of them!	Honey, Stevia, agave nectar, dates and figs, low-sugar fruits (such as apples, pears, kiwi, avocado, strawberries, blueberries, cherries, raspberries and rhubarb); dark chocolate (organic 70%+ cocoa solids); homemade smoothies; fresh homemade juices; water with fresh lemon/lime /orange/ strawberry infusions.	Supermarkets or other health-food stores.
Table Salt	Table salt is bleached and processed, leaving only two minerals (sodium and chloride). Unchecked, these two minerals can imbalance our bodies and lead to high blood pressure.	Pink Himalayan crystal salt, which contains a full spectrum of minerals and trace minerals.	Health-food stores, some supermarkets or online.

 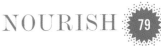

NO-NOS	WHY ELIMINATE	REPLACE WITH	BUY FROM
MSG (monosodium glutamate, a flavour enhancer) Found in a lot of processed and packaged junk foods, such as Doritos, Pringles and Snack-a-Jacks, as well as many Chinese foods.	MSG can lead to headaches and health complications.	Pink Himalayan crystal salt.	Holland & Barrett, Wholefoods, your local health-food store.
Tap Water	Tap water is full of the chemicals we are trying to eradicate from stored fatty tissue!	Filtered water (BRITA or other) or bottled water.	BRITA filters can be found in most supermarket and homewares stores.

Now for the good stuff! Here is a list of all the detoxifying foods to ADD to your diet this week.

ADD	HOW TO TAKE	WHY TAKE	BUY FROM
Clean filtered or bottled water.	Take the amount of water you are currently drinking and double it if you are drinking less than 1 litre per day. N.B. If you are drinking NO water at the moment aim for 1 x 500ml bottle.	Water is the best medium for transporting toxins through the body to be eliminated by the kidneys (through urine) and by the bowels (through your no. 2s).	Filter your own at home or buy from a store.

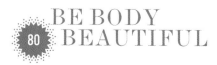

BE BODY
BEAUTIFUL

ADD	HOW TO TAKE	WHY TAKE	BUY FROM
Clean and Clear Smoothie	Follow the recipe for the Clean and Clear Smoothie (page 156) and have at least one per day. Ideal for mid-morning or mid-afternoon when you'd normally want to reach for the sugar!	Green vegetables, in particular broccoli, kale and cabbage, support the liver in processing many toxins.	Ideally buy fresh vegetables from your local greengrocer or arrange for an organic produce delivery to your door. But if your only option is frozen veg, these are fine too.
Additional green vegetables (see fibrous green veg table on page 83)	Consume no fewer than four different green vegetables (raw or steamed) in addition to your Clean and Clear Smoothie every day. You can have these all at once or split across your meals.	Green vegetables not only provide nutrients for detoxification, but also the fibre required to shift toxins and waste through the bowels.	Greengrocers, online organic deliveries or supermarkets.
Herbal teas	Consume at least one cup of herbal tea this week. Choose organic where possible. N.B. Watch for 'flavoured teas' as these may have no active ingredients and contain artificial flavours.	Peppermint, nettle, fennel, liquorice and dandelion teas are all powerful detoxifiers. Green and white teas in particular contain fat-burning nutrients called catechins that help to switch on the fat-burning process.	Health-food stores, tea specialists, supermarkets.

 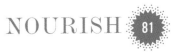

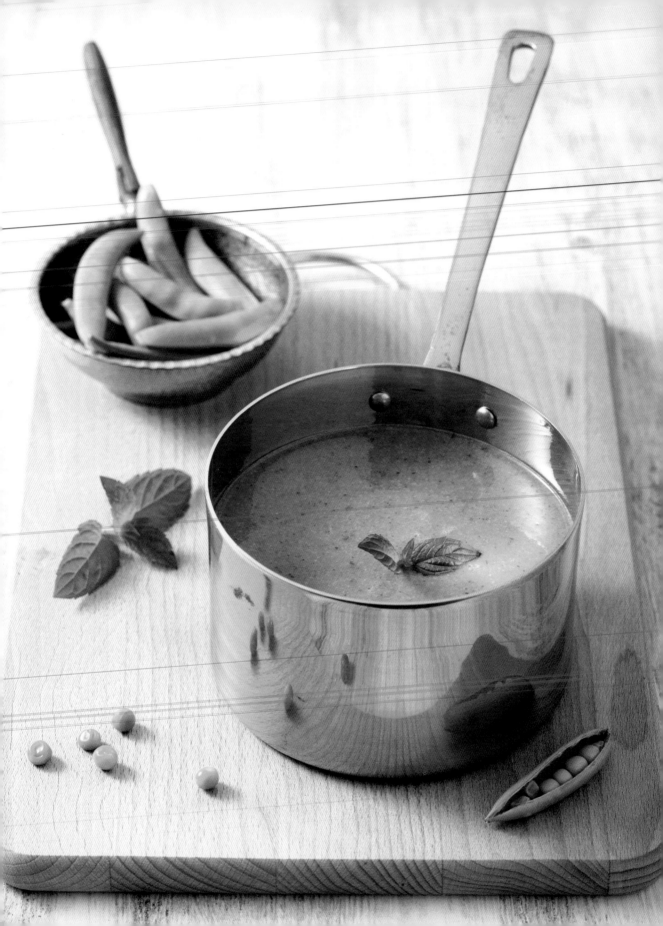

Useful Tables for Week 1

FIBROUS VEGETABLES	DETOX HERBS & TEAS	GOOD FATS	LOW-SUGER FRUITS 1 SERVING = 1 PIECE OR 1/2 CUP
Artichokes	**Herbs:**	**Animal Sources:**	Bananas
Asparagus	Chives	Oily fish	Kiwi
Aubergine	Coriander	Eggs	Green apples
Bamboo shoots	Mint	Butter	Berries
Beansprouts	Parsley	Ghee	Lemons
Beet greens			Limes
Broccoli	Add these to your	**Plant sources (don't**	
Brussels sprouts (what	salads!	**heat/cook with):**	
kind of Christmas		Avocado	
would it be without	**Teas:**	Olive oil	
them!)	Peppermint	Sunflower oil	
Cabbage	Nettle	Nut oils	
Carrots	Fennel	Hemp and flaxseed	
Cauliflower	Liquorice	oils	
Celery	Dandelion		
Courgettes	Green	**Plant sources**	
Cucumber	White	**(may be heated):**	
Fennel		Coconut oil	
Green Beans		Rice bran oil	
Kale		Sesame oil	
Lettuce (all)			
Mangetout			
Mushrooms			
Mustard greens			
Okra			
Pak choi			
Radishes			
Sea vegetables			
(seaweeds such as nori,			
glasswort and			
pickleweed)			
Sugar snap peas			
Spinach			
Spirulina (powder			
or capsules)			
Swiss chard			
Tomatoes			

Love your Greens

Green/fibrous vegetables don't have to be boring or bland!

Add tomatoes, olives and feta cheese to salad greens, dress naturally with balsamic vinegar and olive oil, or just with plain and simple lemon juice.

Melt a little organic butter over steamed greens or drizzle with olive oil, lemon juice and pink Himalayan crystal salt.

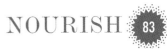

Example Meal Planner for Week 1

N.B. Veggie options have been included for each meal where needed. Have no more than three desserts in any given week, and only choose desserts from our Dessert List (page 106).

UPON WAKING	BREAKFAST	LUNCH	SNACK	EVENING MEAL
DAY 1				
1 pint water with juice of ½ a fresh lemon	Poached eggs and spinach on German rye bread	Green Soup (page 180)/ Hummus and Dippers	Clean and Clear Smoothie (page 156)	Thai Steamed Fish with Asian Greens (page 211) or Lentil Bolognaise (page 197)
DAY 2				
1 pint water with juice of ½ a fresh lemon	Natural Porridge with apple and cinnamon (page 160)	Chicken, Strawberry and Kiwi Salad (page 175) or Superfood Salad (page 169)	Clean and Clear Smoothie	Veggie Chilli with brown rice or quinoa (page 199)
DAY 3				
1 pint water with juice of ½ a fresh lemon	Savoury scramble (page 162) PLUS 1 serving of low-sugar fruit (choose from table on page 83)	Green Soup (page 180)/ Hummus and Dippers	Clean and Clear Smoothie	Greek Meatballs (page 216) and salad or Cauliflower and Chickpea Curry (page 194)
DAY 4				
1 pintwater with juice of ½ a fresh lemon	Berry Medley with Coconut Yogurt (page 221)	Fennel and Walnut Salad (page 167) Green Soup/ Hummus and Dippers	Clean and Clear Smoothie	Healthy Fish Pie (page 217) with a green side salad or Aubergine Cannelloni

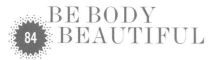

UPON WAKING	BREAKFAST	LUNCH	SNACK	EVENING MEAL
DAY 5 1 pint water with juice of ½ a fresh lemon	Feta, tomato and parsley omelette	Pick 'n' Mix Lunch Salad (page 171)	Clean and Clear Smoothie	RWL Stir-fry with brown rice (page 212)
DAY 6 1 pint water with juice of ½ a fresh lemon	Natural Porridge with banana and desiccated coconut	Sushi Salad (page 172) or Vegetable and Cashew Nori Rolls (page 184)	Clean and Clear Smoothie	Aubergine Cannelloni (page 209) with a side of steamed greens
DAY 7 1 pint water with juice of ½ a fresh lemon	Berry Medley with Coconut Yogurt	Vegetable and Cashew Nori Rolls	Clean and Clear Smoothie	Pacific Island Fish Curry (page 195) with quinoa or Spiced Vegetable Quinoa (page 187)

Other Snack Ideas for the Next Six Weeks

Low-sugar fruits, natural nuts, olives, hummus, vegetable sticks, 'Bounce Balls', boiled eggs, fresh berries, natural yogurt.

 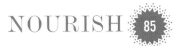

Week 2: 'Add More Antioxidants'

In week 1 you started to eliminate some of the serious no-no foods from your diet. And you've done brilliantly to get these out of your kitchen cupboards and hopefully out of your life for good! There are a few more eliminations this week but, more importantly, your focus this week is to get more ANTIOXIDANTS into your body!

Antioxidants are needed to keep free radicals in check. Free radicals are by-products of metabolism that unless 'neutralized' by an antioxidant will continue to cause tissue and cell damage, leading to inflammation and premature ageing. It is also likely that a major cause of cellulite is free radical damage.

Nutrition Tasks for 'Clean and Clear' Week 2 (days 8–14)

Now for MORE good stuff – maintain week one's ADD-INs as well as the following:

ADD	HOW TO TAKE	WHY TAKE	BUY FROM
Highly antioxidant berries Such as blueberries, raspberries, strawberries and dried goji berries.	Add as part of your meal plans. Great as snacks on their own or in breakfast options, salads or smoothies! Fresh or frozen berries are fine. Wash non-organic products in lemon juice and filtered water to remove pesticide residue.	Antioxidants are important in the detoxification process. They also help our cells to stay youthful, including our skin cells!	Greengrocers, online organic deliveries or supermarkets.

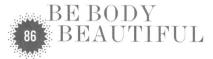

ADD	HOW TO TAKE	WHY TAKE	BUY FROM
Clean proteins (Organic or free-range animal proteins) Such as legumes (all peas, beans and lentils), quinoa, spirulina powder or capsules, naturally fermented/non-GM soya (tofu and tempeh), eggs, poultry, fresh fish, minimal red meat and mixed nuts.	Aim to consume at least one clean protein source at every main meal. Limit all nuts to a handful per day in total. N.B. Quinoa is also a carbohydrate so rely on it more as a carb than protein for this plan. 1 Protein Portion = 150g meat/chicken (approx 1 breast) or 2 eggs or 100g fish (approx. 1 fillet/piece) or 1 cup cooked quinoa/plant proteins or 1–2tsp spirulina	We've already mentioned the importance of protein for supporting skin and muscle health and tone as well as helping to keep blood sugar stable and insulin levels under control.	Supermarkets, butcher's, health-food stores.
Wheat-free 'clean carbohydrates' Such as root vegetables (except white potatoes), oats, rye, spelt, barley, brown rice, quinoa, millet and buckwheat.	You can consume one portion of wheat-free clean carbs at two out of three main meals in a day. Serving size = ½–¾ cup of cooked grains (e.g. rice, buckwheat, oatmeal, etc.) or 1 slice of German rye bread or 1 cup of cooked root vegetables (any one or a mix).	Wheat-free carbs tend to be less processed and have higher levels of nutrition. They also have a slower sugar release into the bloodstream, helping to manage insulin, which plays a role in fat loss.	Supermarkets, health-food stores.

 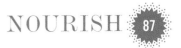

This week's no-nos . . .

In addition to week one's eliminations, this week you also should ELIMINATE:

NO-NOS	WHY ELIMINATE	REPLACE WITH	BUY FROM
Wheat grains/ wheat products Such as conventional bread, pita, wraps, croissants, bagels, pasta (both white and brown), couscous, bulgar wheat, wheat flour, biscuits and cakes – i.e. most bakery items.	Wheat, like many grains, contains a protein called gluten that can cause nutritional deficiency, digestive stress, IBS, skin problems, other allergies and fatigue. Not to mention weight gain and bloating.	Rye, brown or wild rice, pulses and legumes; nut flours instead of wheat flour.	Supermarkets or health-food stores.
Dairy products from cows (except organic butter and plain organic yogurt). These include: cheese, fruit yogurts, sour cream, processed dairy desserts, ice cream, crème fraîche, cream and milk.	Dairy is another high-allergen food, causing unnecessary bloating and lethargy in many people. It's a good idea on detox to keep this out of your diet. You can still have plain organic yogurt (if you are not lactose intolerant) and organic butter.	Almond, rice, oat or hemp milk; feta, goat's or buffalo cheese; plain organic yogurt.	Supermarkets and health-food stores.
Alcohol	Alcohol stresses the liver, stops nutrient absorption and contains empty calories.	Water, chlorophyll water, herbal teas, hot water and lemon, or fruit- and cucumber-infused water.	Health-food stores or supermarkets.

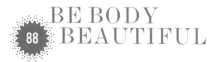

NO-NOS	WHY ELIMINATE	REPLACE WITH	BUY FROM
Coffee and normal tea	Both are stimulants and a stress on the liver. During detox we want the liver focused on detoxing stored toxic fat as opposed to being distracted by other stimulants coming into the system.	Green tea, white tea and liquorice, dandelion, nettle or peppermint herbal teas.	Health-food stores or supermarkets.
Soya 'dairy' Replacements such as soya milk, yogurt and cheese.	These products are processed and very far removed from the original form of natural soya, which may have health-promoting properties. But in this refined, genetically modified and chemically enhanced form, soya may have negative effects on the thyroid gland.	Oat, rice or almond milk; goat's milk and yogurt; goat's and sheep's cheeses.	Supermarkets.
'Cheat' carbohydrates	These are generally wheat-based, highly processed and highly refined sugary or starchy foods. Some, like white potatoes, are purely categorized as 'cheats' because they cause a high level of insulin production.	Wheat-free clean carbs (see list on page 90).	Health-food stores or supermarkets.

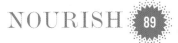

Useful Tables for Week 2

NO-NOS CHEAT CARBOHYDRATES	WHEAT-FREE CLEAN CARBOHYDRATES	CLEAN PROTEINS
White potatoes	Sweet potatoes	**Animal Sources:**
Potato cakes	Butternut squash	Fish
Wheat pasta (white and brown)	Parsnips	Eggs
Couscous	Swede	Poultry (chicken, turkey)
Wheat bread	Yams	Game
Bread rolls	Turnip	Red meat
Crumpets	Celeriac	
Muffins	Brown rice	**Plant:**
Bakery items such as cakes,	Wild rice	Spirulina
pastries, bagels	Buckwheat	Beans
White sugar	Quinoa	Peas
Brown sugar	Millet	Legumes
Synthetic honey	Oatmeal/rolled oats	Quinoa
Golden syrup	German rye bread	
	Gluten-free pasta	
	Manuka honey	
	Raw organic honey	
	Stevia	

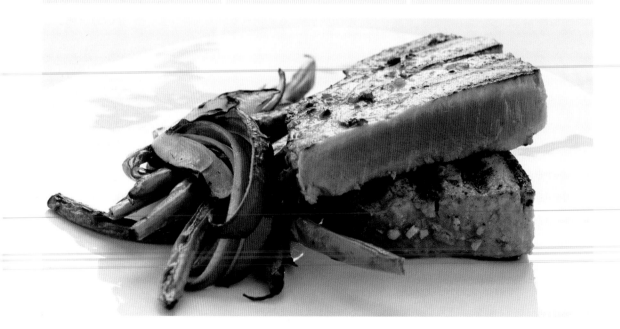

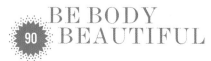

Example Meal Planner for Week 2

N.B. Have no more than three desserts in any given week, and only choose desserts from our Dessert List (page 106).

UPON WAKING	BREAKFAST	LUNCH	SNACK	EVENING MEAL
DAY 1 1 pint water with juice of ½ a fresh lemon	Sticky Egg and Avocado Salad (page 168)	Asparagus and Artichoke Soup (page 177)	Antioxidant Blend (page 158)	Pea and Parsley Crepe (page 186)
DAY 2 1 pint water with juice of ½ a fresh lemon	Fruity Quinoa with Home-roasted Almonds (page 163)	Salmon Nori Rolls (page 184) or Beetroot and Egg Salad (page 167)	Antioxidant Blend	Tarragon Turkey Burgers (page 200) with a mix of steamed greens or mixed salad or Cannellini Bean and Quinoa Patties (page 189) with mixed steamed greens
DAY 3 1 pint water with juice of ½ a fresh lemon	Coconut Berry Salad (page 161)	Superfood Salad (add chicken if you like) (page 169)	Antioxidant Blend	Beef and Tomato Coconut Curry (page 193) served with buckwheat and raw baby spinach or Spiced Chickpea Casserole (page 206) on a bed of baby spinach

 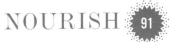

UPON WAKING	BREAKFAST	LUNCH	SNACK	EVENING MEAL
DAY 4 1 pint water with juice of ½ a fresh lemon	Sticky Egg and Avocado Salad	Asparagus and Artichoke Soup	Antioxidant Blend	Leftover Beef and Tomato Coconut Curry (as day 3, no buckwheat) on baby spinach
DAY 5 1 pint water with juice of ½ a fresh lemon	Fruity Quinoa with Home-roasted Almonds	Fennel Mixed Salad (page 170)	Antioxidant Blend	Three Bean Chilli served on brown rice and a thick layer of raw baby spinach or wilted kale
DAY 6 1 pint water with juice of ½ a fresh lemon	Coconut Berry Salad	Asparagus and Artichoke Soup	Antioxidant Blend	Leftover Three Bean Chilli (as day 5, no brown rice)
DAY 7 1 pint water with juice of ½ a fresh lemon	Sticky Eggs and Avocado Salad on German Rye toast	Superfood Salad (add chicken if you like)	Antioxidant Blend	Pea and Parsley Crepe

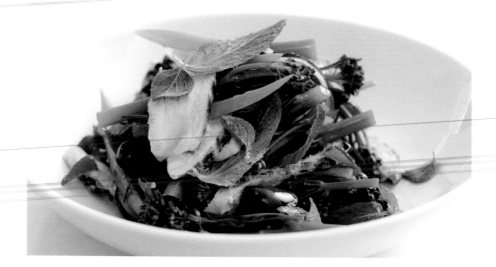

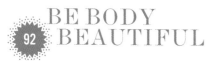

Week 3: 'Wobble Wipeout'

So … the nutrition tasks outlined this far are capable of getting you GOOD results on your fat-busting mission, but we don't just want you to get good results, we want you to get GREAT results! Therefore it's time to step up your detox by eliminating just a couple more foods from your diet …

Nutrition Tasks for 'Clean and Clear' Week 3 (days 15–21)

Eliminate the following in addition to those eliminations in weeks one and two.

NO-NOS	WHY ELIMINATE	REPLACE WITH	BUY FROM
Red meat and pork	Heavy meats can be hard to digest. During detox the best results are gained when the digestive system gets a bit of a rest from incoming stresses.	Poultry, fish, organic eggs. Some people prefer to go vegetarian through detox, but it is still important to get all your proteins from spirulina and pulses.	Supermarkets, health-food stores, butchers and farmers' markets.
Gluten grains (except rye and oats) This list includes: corn, spelt and barley.	Most people digest food better and feel less bloated when off wheat and gluten. For detox it's important to keep these out of the diet.	Non-gluten grains, such as quinoa, brown rice, buckwheat, amaranth and millet, as well as colourful starchy vegetables – squash, sweet potatoes, carrots, parsnips and swede.	Supermarkets, greengrocers or health-food stores.

 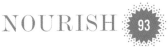

Example Meal Planner for Week 3

N.B. Have no more than three desserts in any given week, and only choose desserts from our Dessert List (page 106).

UPON WAKING	BREAKFAST	LUNCH	SNACK	EVENING MEAL
DAY 1				
Antioxidant Blend (page 158)	Almond and Date Smoothie (page 154)	Lettuce Chicken Tacos (page 208)	Clean and Clear Smoothie (page 156)	Healthy Fish Pie (page 217)
DAY 2				
Antioxidant Blend	Natural Porridge with cinnamon and honey (page 160)	Feel-good Veggie Soup (page 182)	Clean and Clear Smoothie	Black Bean Patties (page 205)
DAY 3				
Antioxidant Blend	BLAT (beetroot, lettuce, avocado and tomato) stacked on German rye bread	Green salad with sliced avocado, green beans and lemon	Clean and Clear Smoothie	RWL Stir-fry on brown rice or quinoa (page 212)
DAY 4				
Antioxidant Blend	Breakfast 'Roughie' (page 162)	Feel-good Veggie Soup	Clean and Clear Smoothie	Thai Steamed Fish with Asian Greens (page 211)
DAY 5				
Antioxidant Blend	Feta, tomato and parsley omelette	Feel-good Veggie Soup	Clean and Clear Smoothie	Garlic Rosemary Lamb Chops (page 214) with roasted sweet potato and steamed greens
DAY 6				
Antioxidant Blend	Natural Porridge with cinnamon and honey	Beetroot and Egg Salad (page 167)	Clean and Clear Smoothie	Grilled chicken breast with green salad
DAY 7				
Antioxidant Blend	Almond and Date Smoothie (page 154)	Lettuce Chicken Tacos	Clean and Clear Smoothie	Pacific Island Fish Curry with steamed greens (page 195)

BE BODY BEAUTIFUL

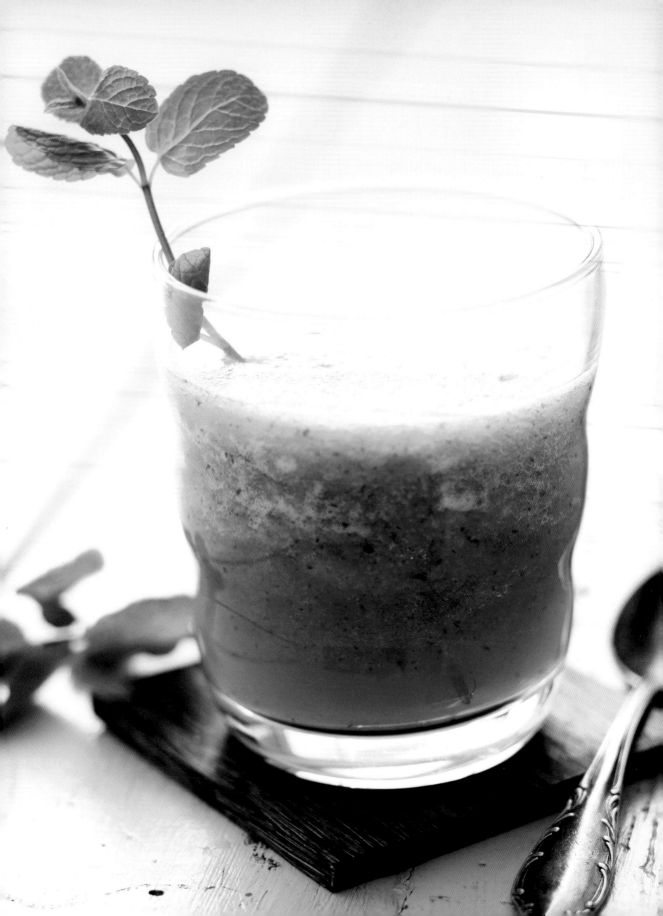

THE PLAN: STEP 2 – NOURISH AND REPAIR (WEEKS 4–6)

Week 4: 'Sup'ed Up'

Well done for doing so well on Step 1… Detoxing is never easy, but you have done brilliantly! Now we are on to the equally important Step 2. This 'Nourish and Repair' phase is crucial for turning orange-peel-looking skin into smoother, more toned-looking model material. So this week we are focused on using superfoods and their 'Sup'ed Up' nutrient content to provide the raw materials to support the collagen and elastin properties of your skin.

Nutrition Tasks for 'Nourish and Repair' Week 4 (days 22–28)

Maintain the previous weeks' ADD-INs as well as including these superfoods!

ADD	HOW TO TAKE	WHY TAKE	BUY FROM
Maca Powder (maca is a root belonging to the radish family)	Add to smoothies and use to make the Maca Dip (page 182) as a delicious snack or part of a breakfast.	Maca powder is considered a superfood, helping to balance hormones and detoxify the body.	Health-food stores or online
Ground Flaxseeds	Add to your smoothies, breakfast options, yogurt and berries, or simply take in water.	Ground flaxseeds are a great source of essential fats for healthy skin as well as being full of detoxifying fibre!	Health-food stores or online

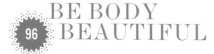

ADD	HOW TO TAKE	WHY TAKE	BUY FROM
Chia Seeds	Add these to your breakfasts and smoothies too! Or you can simply take them in water.	Chia seeds are high in essential oils that keep our skin cells taut and youthful. They are also very cleansing on the digestive system. Also, like flaxseeds, they act as a 'mop' for toxic hormonal waste in the bowels.	Health-food stores or online.
Raw Cocoa Nibs	Add these to your smoothies, breakfast options or simply snack on them as they come. Be prepared though: the high tannin component makes them really bitter – the more bitter, the better!	Raw cocoa is the most antioxidant food on the planet. Bursting with beauty minerals such as iron, zinc and manganese, this is a must for healthy skin!	Health-food stores or online.

Example Meal Planner for Week 4

N.B. Have no more than three desserts in any given week, and only choose desserts from our Dessert List (page 106).

UPON WAKING	BREAKFAST	LUNCH	SNACK	EVENING MEAL
DAY 1 1 pint water with juice of ½ a fresh lemon	7 Superfoods Cereal (page 164)	Beetroot and Egg Salad (page 167)	½ cup Maca Dip (page 182) with green apple slices	Steamed Mediterranean Cod (page 190) or Spiced Vegetable Quinoa (page 187) with salad or green vegetables

 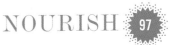

UPON WAKING	BREAKFAST	LUNCH	SNACK	EVENING MEAL
DAY 2 1 pint water with juice of ½ a fresh lemon	Almond Milk Smoothie (page 154)	Carrot, Cashew and Chilli Soup (page 176)	Magic Magic Maca Smoothie (page 158)	Spiced Vegetable Quinoa with leafy green salad
DAY 3 1 pint water with juice of ½ a fresh lemon	Sticky Eggs and Avocado Salad on Rye Bread (page 168)	Paleo Plate (page 187)	Clean and Clear Smoothie (page 156)	Beef and Tomato Coconut Curry (page 193) with wilted spinach or Basic Dhal (page 204) with wilted spinach
DAY 4 1 pint water with juice of ½ a fresh lemon	Malibu Beach Smoothie (page 154)	Carrot, Cashew and Chilli Soup	½ cup Maca Dip with green apple slices	Leftover Beef and Tomato Curry with a mix of steamed greens or Lentil Bolognaise (page 197)
DAY 5 1 pint water with juice of ½ a fresh lemon	7 Superfoods Cereal	Beetroot and Egg Salad	Magic Maca Smoothie	Grilled Mackerel Fillets with Apple Chutney (page 202) and a mix of steamed greens or Cauliflower and Chickpea Curry (page 194)
DAY 6 1 pint water with juice of ½ a fresh lemon	Banana Berry Smoothie (page 156)	Carrot, Cashew and Chilli Soup	Clean and Clear Smoothie	Savoury Scramble (page 162)
DAY 7 1 pint water with juice of ½ a fresh lemon	7 Superfoods Cereal	Beetroot and Egg Salad	Clean and Clear Smoothie	Superfood Salad (page 163) (with chicken or fish if you like)

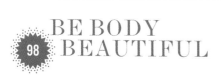

Week 5: 'Skin Food'

Is it possible that if I mention the word ANTIOXIDANTS one more time, you might just explode? I've certainly banged on about these little beauties a number of times now in this plan, but there is a reason they feature so often and that is because they are super, super, super important in this two-fold approach to burning body fat and eradicating cellulite.

1. They help skin cells to stay smooth and taut.
2. They help clear your fat cells of toxins.
This week I want to introduce to you the antioxidant (yes there it is again) silica – also known as silicon dioxide.

Silica

Whenever collagen fibres (the structural components of skin and all soft tissue) are damaged by free radicals, silica is required to rebuild and regenerate our skin tissue, by enhancing collagen production. Quite conveniently silica is also great for removing toxins stored in and under the skin (i.e. cellulite!)

More on Omega-3 for Great Skin

Omega-3 is the most deficient essential fatty acid in the diet of the western world and yet it's the one that we probably need the most, especially when it comes to a) fat BURNING and b) skin health!

Deemed 'essential' because we cannot make this fatty acid ourselves, we HAVE to get it from our diet. Oily fish, eggs, chia and flaxseeds are great sources of omega-3; however, to get optimal levels into our bodies we would have to consume around twenty-four servings of oily fish every week! That is just INSANE – surely no one likes fish that much!

Omega-3 signals to the body to switch ON your fat-burning enzymes and switch OFF your fat-storing enzymes (reason alone to take this powerful 'super fat')! It also helps to maintain the integrity of your skin cells – keeping them looking healthy.

 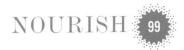

You can get omega-3 naturally through eating the foods listed above, but I also recommend taking a high-quality omega-3 supplement on top of these.

Nutrition Tasks for 'Nourish and Repair' Week 5 (days 29–35)

Continue to follow your detox food eliminations and water intake from weeks three and four but now focus on high-silica foods such as rosemary, alfalfa, romaine lettuce, spinach, burdock root, radishes, cucumber, capsicums (sweet peppers), tomatoes and oats.

Example Meal Planner for Week 5

N.B. Have no more than three desserts, and only from the Dessert List (page 106).

UPON WAKING	BREAKFAST	LUNCH	SNACK	EVENING MEAL
DAY 1 Antioxidant Blend	Breakfast 'Roughie' (page 162)	Beauty Bowl (page 207)	½ cup Maca Dip with green apple slices (page 182)	Thai Fish Soup (page 178) or Spiced Vegetable Quinoa (page 187)
DAY 2 Antioxidant Blend	Green Goddess Smoothie (page 153)	Carrot and Coriander Soup (page 180) with Hummus and Dippers	Magic Maca Smoothie (page 158)	Cauliflower and Chickpea Curry (page 194) on a bed of steamed green veg
DAY 3 Antioxidant Blend	Natural Porridge with mixed berries and squeezy honey (page 160)	Seaweed Rolls (page 186) or Vegetable and Cashew Nori Rolls (page 184)	Clean and Clear Smoothie (page 156)	Grilled chicken breast with Greek salad or Cannellini Bean and Quinoa Patties (page 189)

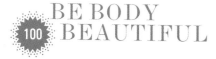

Be Body BEAUTIFUL

UPON WAKING	BREAKFAST	LUNCH	SNACK	EVENING MEAL
DAY 4 Antioxidant Blend	Fresh Fruit with Raw Nut Cream (page 221)	Carrot and Coriander Soup with Hummus and Dippers	½ cup Maca Dip with green apple slices	Salmon with Olive and Garlic Sauce (page 215) served with steamed greens or Cauliflower and Chickpea Curry
DAY 5 Antioxidant Blend	Green Goddess Smoothie (page 153)	Quinoa Tabbouleh (page 207)	Magic Maca Smoothie	RWL Stir-fry (page 212) on brown rice noodles (optional) or Veggie Chilli (page 199)
DAY 6 Antioxidant Blend	Berry Medley with Coconut Yogurt (page 221)	Carrot and Coriander Soup with Hummus & Dippers	Clean and Clear Smoothie	Lentil Bolognaise (page 197) with a side of seasonal veg
DAY 7 Antioxidant Blend	Purple Porridge (page 161)	Salmon Nori Rolls (page 184) or Vegetable and Cashew Nori Rolls	Clean and Clear Smoothie	Basic Dhal with vegetables and brown rice (page 204)

'FOLLOW THIS PLAN
AND YOU WILL FEEL
REVITALIZED,
HAPPY AND HEALTHY.'

 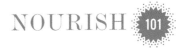

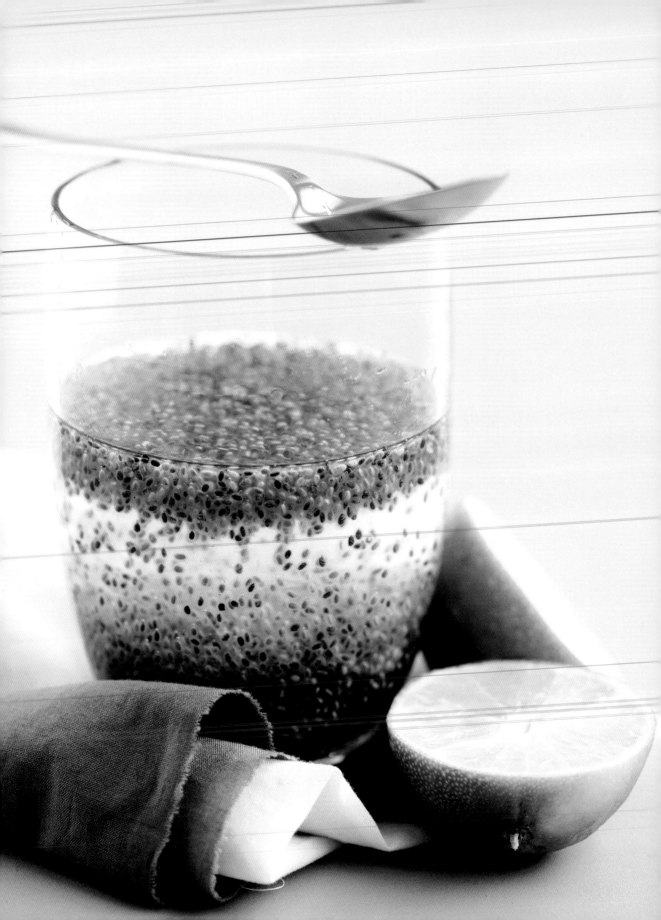

Week 6: 'Model Material'

Wow, girls! You've got body beautiful in (nearly) six weeks. Congratulations, you are almost done!

This week, we really want you to keep up all the fabulous food changes you have made over the past five weeks and not just for this last week! If you can continue with the following checklist for as long as possible you'll continue to feel revitalized, happy and healthy. Remember, this is a lifestyle choice and it's long-term, not a short-term fix.

Maintenance Checklist

Remember the F.E.M. formula (food, exercise, massage).

• Food

Make Fibrous Vegetables Your Food Focus

Aim for a MINIMUM of 7 but up to 11 different servings of fibrous veg per day. By making the bulk of your meals vegetable-based, you will never have to worry about hitting this target. Salads are the simplest and most efficient way to get these into you. Smoothies are also a great way to cram lots of vegetables and low-sugar fruits into one meal!

• *Stay Well Hydrated*

Drink at least 2–3 litres of clean filtered or bottled water every day – always starting the day with a large pint of either chlorophyll or fresh lemon to kick-start a daily cleanse.

• *Highly Antioxidant Foods*

Continue to consume antioxidants at every meal and throughout the day. Your skin will thank you for it! These include:

★ Berries
★ Catechins (found in green and white teas – aim for 3 cups per day)
★ Vitamin C (from fruits and green vegetables)
★ Vitamin E and selenium (a good source is Brazil nuts)

 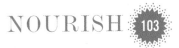

* Vitamin A (found in carrots)
* Silica
* Rosemary
* Raw cocoa
* Chia seeds
* Maca powder

Consume at least once a day either an Antioxidant Blend super cellulite-busting drink or a Clean and Clear Smoothie.

• *Clean Carbs*

Eat 1–2 portions of clean carbs per day. Do this for five out of the seven days in a week. Then try and go totally carb free for two non-consecutive days each week.

• *Keep Cheat Foods to a Minimum*

Consume the following 'cheat' foods no more than once every fortnight:

* Wheat
* Processed bakery goods
* Dairy products from cows (except plain unsweetened organic yogurt)
* Alcohol
* Sugar
* Soya 'dairy' products

And these ones no more than once a week:

* Coffee
* Normal tea

• *Never Again 'No-nos'*

Eliminate margarine and foods and products containing aspartame and MSG (monosodium glutamate) from your diet for ever.

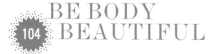

• Exercise

Continue to exercise at least 3-4 times per week, performing a range of metabolic training exercises – like those in the Exercise at Home and Exercise in the Park routines (pages 139–46).

• Massage

Try to have regular lymphatic drainage massages if you can, but definitely make sure you dry body brush every day! Remember to brush the skin of areas affected by cellulite towards the heart because that is the way our circulation naturally flows, so brushing toxins into circulation to be processed is more effective.

Example Meal Planner for Week 6

N.B. Have no more than three desserts in any given week, and only choose desserts from our Dessert List (page 106).

UPON WAKING	BREAKFAST	LUNCH	SNACK	EVENING MEAL
DAY 1 1 pint water with juice of ½ a fresh lemon	Purple Porridge (page 161)	Avocado, Tomato and Sliced Mozzarella Salad	½ cup Maca Dip with green apple slices (page 182)	Salmon with Olive and Garlic Sauce and vegetables (page 215) or Pea and Parsley Crepe (page 186)
DAY 2 Antioxidant Blend (page 158)	Green Goddess Smoothie (page 153)	Hearty Vegetable Soup (page 178) with German rye bread or buckwheat	Magic Maca Smoothie (page 158)	Homemade Beef Bolognaise (page 203) or Lentil Bolognaise (page 197) on a bed of wilted spinach
DAY 3 1 pint water with juice of ½ a fresh lemon	Smoked salmon and avocado slices	Beetroot and Egg Salad (page 167)	Clean and Clear Smoothie (page 156)	Turkey and Chickpea Curry (page 190) or Cauliflower snd Chickpea Curry (page 194)

UPON WAKING	BREAKFAST	LUNCH	SNACK	EVENING MEAL
DAY 4 Antioxidant Blend	Sticky Egg and Avocado Salad (page 168)	Salmon Nori Rolls (page 184) or Vegetable and Cashew Nori Rolls (page 184)	½ cup Maca Dip with green apple slices	Parsnip Curry served on buckwheat and a bed of baby spinach
DAY 5 1 pint water with juice of ½ a fresh lemon	Fruity Quinoa with Home-Roasted Almonds (page 163)	Grain-free Superfood Salad Spiced Vegetable Quinoa (page 169)	Magic Maca Smoothie	Hearty Vegetable Soup followed by Grilled Chicken Skewers or Spiced Vegetable Quinoa with mixed steamed greens
DAY 6 Antioxidant Blend	Green Goddess Smoothie	Hearty Vegetable Soup and	Clean and Clear Smoothie	Chickpea and Parsnip Curry (add chicken, prawns or tofu if you like) served on a bed of baby spinach and/or beansprouts (page 192)
DAY 7 1 pint water with juice of ½ a fresh lemon	Savoury Scramble (page 162)	Superfood Salad	Clean and Clear Smoothie	Steamed Mediterranean Cod with mixed steamed veg (page 190) or Pea and Parsley Crepe (page 186) or RWL Stir-fry (page 212) (add prawns, scallops or chicken if you like) served with brown rice

Dessert List
★ Avocado, Chocolate & Strawberry Mousse (page 218)
★ Berry Crunch (page 223)
★ Berry Medley with Coconut Yogurt (page 221)
★ Chia Seed Pudding (page 222)
★ Dark Chocolate Shake (page 220)
★ Lemon Sorbet (page 220)
★ Yogurt with Passion Fruit & Macadamia Nuts (page 218)

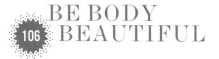

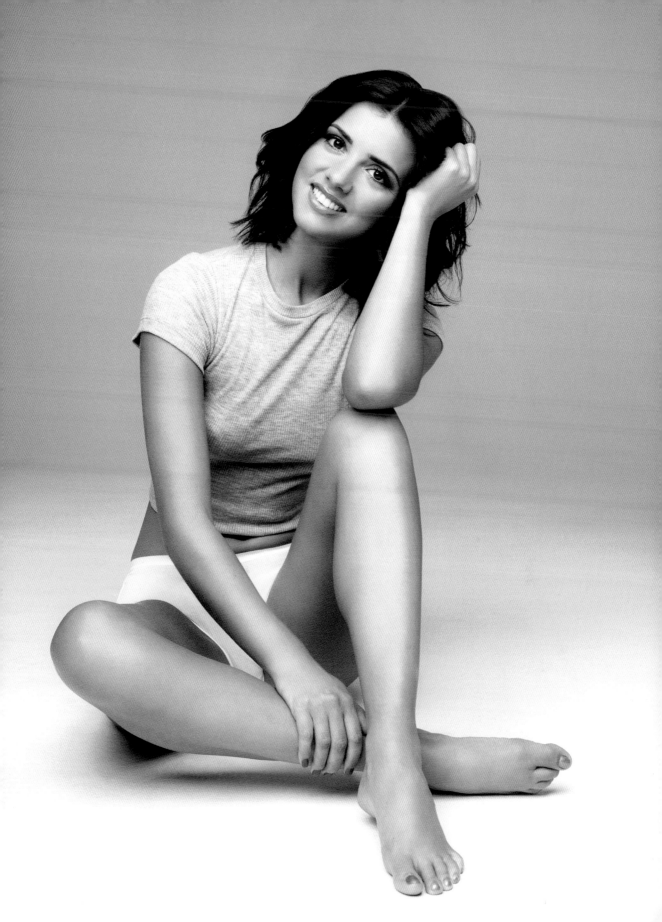

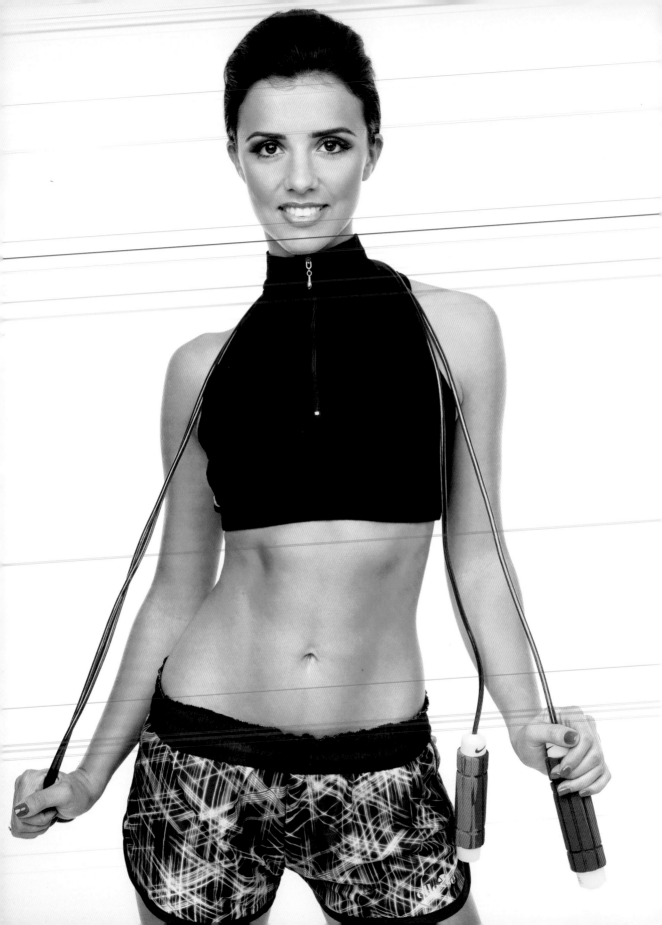

4 ENERGIZE

GET RESULTS WITH LUCY: EXERCISE

My main aim is for this book to reach people who may have gone through similar experiences to me or, if they haven't, to be able to identify with some of the reasons why it's so hard to change the habits of a lifetime. By its very definition, a habit is difficult to break, but once it has been broken there is no turning back – I truly believe that. Exercise needs to become a habit, in the same way as going to the pub every Friday night. It's something that needs to be incorporated into your life so that if you don't do it you will miss it. For those of you that don't already exercise then it's a habit that needs to be created.

I am incredibly passionate and have very strong opinions when it comes to getting fit and I really believe that children should be encouraged to exercise right from a young age. Getting them outside in the fresh air and running around a park is key to their development. I love what Jamie Oliver has tried to introduce with all the healthy eating in schools because it is all about educating people. I really believe that half of the time people don't know that what they are doing is wrong or is detrimental to their children's health. I'm not suggesting for a minute that at parties kids shouldn't have chicken nuggets and sausage rolls, but processed food every day is SO bad for you. The sooner children are introduced to healthy food the more likely they are to embrace it.

I get quite annoyed and frustrated with the number of people who seem to ignore what campaigners like Jamie are trying to do. It's crazy and in my opinion very ignorant. We have so many children who are obese at such a young age and it's awful. I think it's a form of abuse, I really do. Kids don't understand yet but their parents have a duty to make sure they have a balanced healthy diet as well as making sure that they get out and about, whether it's to the park or a swimming lesson. A lot of people say that it's easier

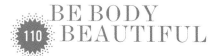

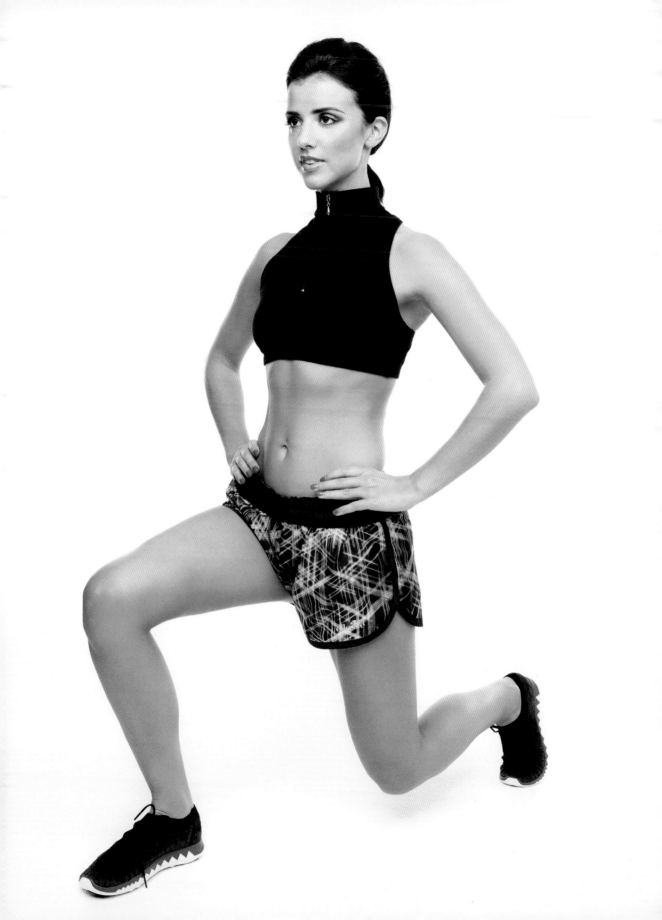

financially for them to buy processed food but buying fresh vegetables and meat really isn't any more expensive and, if you can batch-cook meals, even better! Supermarkets always have special offers on so take advantage of those offers. There are a lot of options when you cook your own food and if your kids do like chicken nuggets or burgers, then why not make them yourself? That way you know exactly what's going into them and I can guarantee that the ingredients won't include teaspoons of sugar! You'd be pretty horrified if you knew what was really in all that processed food and what it can do to your body.

One day I would love to be able to help educate parents about the best diet for their children. People like Annabel Karmel have been amazingly successful and I'd really love to be able to give something back in that sense. I've learnt so much about food and nutritional goodness and how to shop creatively and turn meals around easily. It frustrates me that we don't all know how to do that and we should. It would be a dream come true for me if I could help schools and parents across the country to serve their children healthy, balanced meals that don't cost the world – they just require a teeny tiny bit more time. I'd love to go around schools and teach children about exercise and nutrition in a fun way so that they absorb the message. I'm not claiming to know everything about children, of course I don't! But it really upsets me when I see kids eating the wrong things and carrying weight they don't need and behaving badly because of all the additives they're pumped with. To me, children are really innocent and they should be allowed to be healthy and given a chance. Every child deserves that, no matter what family they are born into.

◦• ◄◦• •◦ • ◦• ◄◦ •◦

I've talked a lot about my body and exercise and since I really properly started to train, it's changed me as a person. I am very different from who I was, even five years ago. When I felt sad about what was happening in my personal life, going to train was the one thing that got me out of the house. It got me up and it focused me.

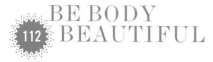

Quite often when you are feeling down and your self-esteem is low you need to focus on something specific and what better thing to focus on than fitness and getting yourself back to having a healthy mind? When you exercise you clear your mind. It's an automatic boost and natural pick-me-up.

I don't think of exercise as a chore any more – it is something that if I didn't do I would miss. If any of you reading this hate the thought of exercise I wish I could tell you how much it doesn't need to be a chore! It's my passion and has got me though some tough times.

Everyone knows how it feels to look in the mirror and hate what they see looking back at them. I defy anyone to say that they have never felt like that at some point in their life. Self-esteem is key to feeling good and loving yourself. My self-esteem was very low following my relationship with Mario. I'd always had a size 32D bust but losing weight had meant that that had disappeared a bit and the fact he'd noticed was like a knife in my heart. It was awful. I can remember him pointing it out to me and it really hurt. That knocked me for a while but I picked myself up and got on with my life. It was always going to go one of two ways and fortunately for me I am a pretty feisty and determined person. I thought, 'Even if you're right, you're a bastard for saying it!' When I want to do something, I do it. There's no stopping me. Hearing that from him made me do something about my body. I needed to get my self-esteem back and learn to appreciate my body once again.

Our bodies are SO important and if we don't look after them, how can they look after us? Very soon after I started properly training I began to see the difference exercise was making and once I started to like what I saw then that spurred me on to do more. You'll find it's the same for you – I promise! The pain threshold is something that you also have to work through. At first you might be totally out of breath in the first five minutes but don't give up because each week you will become fitter and fitter and barriers will be broken. It's not just physically that you feel better either. My mindset was changing. I was becoming a stronger person and I was becoming happier. My

 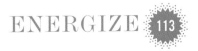

skin was good; I used to suffer from headaches but they were almost non-existent after a couple of weeks of exercise. It was literally down to the training and my diet. They were making such a massive difference to me. I was brighter, bubblier and definitely less moody!

Most recently I have been training for the BBC celebrity gymnastics programme *Tumble*. It's the hardest thing I have EVER done in my life. Gruelling hours spent in the gym working on different gymnastic routines put me right out of my usual comfort zone. So many days I was left in tears thinking, 'I just can't do this!' One time I hurt myself so badly. I was trying to do a front somersault and I managed to kick myself in the eye. It bruised straight away and I looked like I'd been in a fight. On more than one occasion I struggled to get the discipline and I was petrified of the vault. But something inside you gives you determination to succeed and that, along with my coach Katie, who is one of the most determined people I've met, and Billy, my pro partner, got me through. And honestly, I had the most amazing experience of my life. Let's face it, nothing rewarding in life comes easy.

Tumble is the first prime-time show that I have been a part of and it was a big deal for me. It was also the first time that I've properly been on TV since *TOWIE* so I felt incredibly nervous about it all. I knew I'd be wearing tight clothes like leotards and everyone would be having their say, so I wanted to look my best. The moment the show went live, it dawned on me what a big thing I'd embarked on. I thought at any moment I was going to throw up all over the floor! I've never experienced anything like it. The adrenalin, the nerves and the competitive side that I'd never realised I had. All of those emotions mixed into one – it was unbelievable. I'm sure any girl faced with the prospect of being on live TV wearing just a leotard would feel the same, right?

It's hard not to be at your peak of fitness doing a show like *Tumble* because the training schedules were so gruelling. Some days I used to be up at 4am and training by 5am. Then I'd finish at 12.30pm, go to Elstree (where the show was filmed) and not get home until about

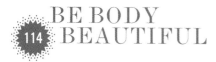

BE BODY
BEAUTIFUL

8pm. It was so hardcore. I'd be lying if I didn't say that there were times when I felt like packing it all in, but that was usually when I was totally knackered – I didn't ever truly think I'd walk out because I was enjoying it and I felt honoured to be involved. If I'd been voted off, honestly I would have been devastated. I wanted it probably more than anyone on the show; but that's not to say I deserved it more. Doing *Tumble* was tough, but it was rewarding. I've got to thank Katie Richards, my coach, who got me through each week. She has an amazing quality of understanding and she totally got me. She knew exactly where my headspace was and was always on hand telling me when I needed to focus, when I was being irrational, when I needed to work harder. That honesty and understanding really helped me because when you are doing hours like that you can become pretty ratty at times. Katie would, in a way, stop me from getting like that. And, of course, my body changing and getting leaner and stronger made it all a bit easier to swallow. It was good to look in the mirror and see what the hardcore training was doing for me. I felt healthy, toned and fulfilled.

There were a few of us on the show that got close. You spend a heap of time with each other so you do end up becoming good mates. I got on really well with Amelle. She's such a lovely girl and she was always smiling. No matter about the early starts and the difficult routines, she always put on a smile. Seriously, I don't know how she did it! I became good mates with Sarah Harding too. I didn't know loads about her, only what I'd read in newspapers and that, but I think she is really misunderstood. She doesn't think she's a cut above, despite being in one of the biggest girl bands ever and she takes a real interest in your life. She's good fun and kind and really different to how I imagined. Us three really stuck together and because we spent so much time with each other we became a bit like a family, helping each other through. If any of us felt low, we would be there to pick them up. I absolutely love Carl Froch the boxer – he is brilliant. He is such a family man and he adores his kids. He was brilliant fun to be around and would always make me laugh.

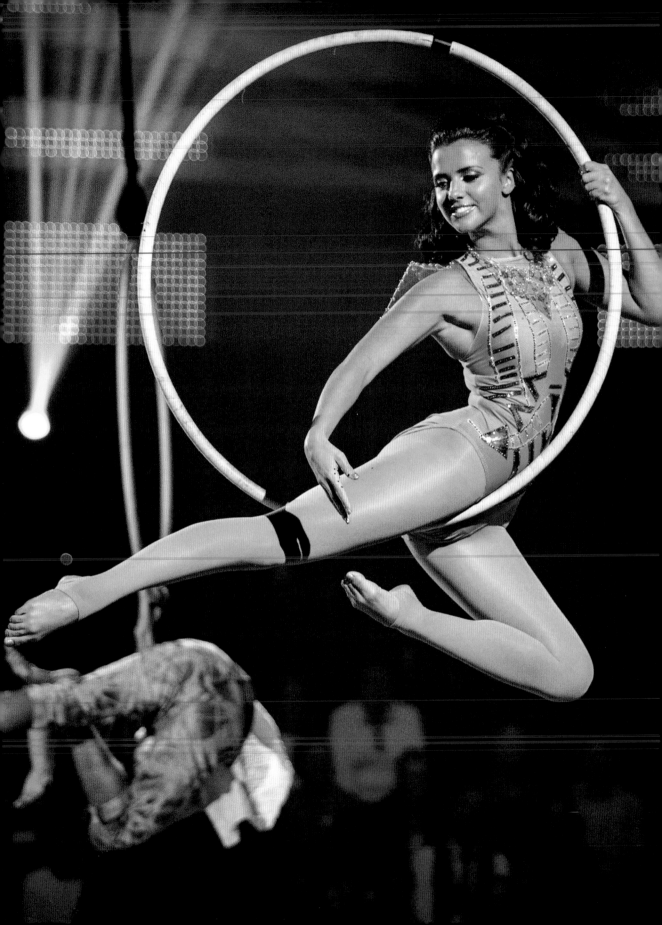

I did loads of routines but I think my favourite was probably the one with the aerial hoop when I was Tinkerbell. I think that was my turning point in the show because I'd had such a bad time in week one when I came bottom of the board and I felt crap about it. I hate failing and that made me feel like a failure. When I got through I wanted to prove that I should be there and that I was good enough to be there. Thank God, by week two I'd changed all the judges' minds. That was 'Tinkerbell week' and I just thought if I'm going out then I'm going out with a bang. Having said all that I did love my prom dress outfit, probably because it reminded me of my own school prom. You get to be so glam and after a week of knocking your body to bits and being bruised all over it's nice to be made-up and look a bit glitzy!

My partner, Billy George, was amazing and supportive and we became really good friends. We were spending pretty much every waking moment together so when the show ended it was weird him not being around me all of the time. It was like having withdrawal symptoms. There were a few stories in the media that suggested that there was something going on, but there wasn't! I think shows like this have got a bit of a reputation because of *Strictly,* but although I was spending a lot of time with Billy training that was all there was to it! We both enjoyed a bit of banter, but as mates. Nothing more. Billy is literally like my annoying, hyperactive little brother. I adore him and I made a friend for life.

We just laughed it off and joked about it, and actually I had just started seeing someone else at the time. I don't want to talk about that much as it is such a new thing, but now, as the book goes to press, I'm really happy.

My body changed hugely on the show – with that amount of training it had to – and when it all ended I wanted to try and keep those parts of my body that I really liked. My bum was a new addition and I loved having it so I've tried really hard to keep that. But I think gymnastics is the only thing that can keep my bum plump and peachy so I'll have to keep it up just for that! Gymnastics must be Kim Kardashian's secret!

Although I want to keep training in gymnastics, it's unsustainable for me to continue doing that level of training. Aside from anything else I am busy with my business and that part of my life was a bit on hold while I trained for *Tumble*. I couldn't run bootycamps and all the things I like to offer so, since the show, I've got stuck back into the business and it's keeping me busy and stopping me from missing *Tumble* too much! I also threw myself into the next big beauty project for me – my own perfume, which I'd been working on for months. I adored the launch party we threw for it. As it's called Wings, and is all about me spreading mine and growing up and becoming a young woman, I made the theme of the party butterflies and wore an amazing dress. It was one of the best nights of my working life and I love seeing the bottle on my dressing table with its beautiful white butterfly wings. Growing up I never thought I'd have my own perfume and it was a dream come true. I've also been busy working on designs for my new range with Ellesse. It's still so weird seeing myself on ad campaigns, I have to pinch myself!

· · · · · · · · · · · ·

Cecilia Harris is my business partner and I have to thank her for giving me a huge amount of support – not just with the business but in every area of my life. She was the person who, alongside Emma, got me healthy and made me realise there was so much more to life. They both helped to re-educate me but Cecilia and her husband Frank are both personal trainers and have always achieved amazing results. They are a huge part of my life and we are great friends. Cecilia – my nutty French trainer who gets her sayings all mixed up and makes me laugh every day – took me in hand and I have never looked back. I thought it was important to hear from Cecilia in this book because she can speak with real authority. What she doesn't know about exercise and getting people into their best shape basically isn't worth knowing. Cecilia will also tell you about the person she saw when she first met me, and the journey we embarked on. Over to you, Cecilia…

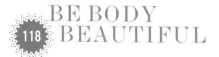

It was January 2013 when I received a call from a friend of mine who runs a local beautician's called Ace in Essex. Sarah asked me if I would like to train Lucy Mecklenburgh.

I didn't really know who Lucy was so I quickly googled her name! I knew she was on *TOWIE* – that was about it – but either way my response would have been yes. Sarah told me that Lucy wanted to get rid of her cellulite and get fit. Having seen pictures of Lucy I found it hard to believe that she had any orange peel but Sarah said Lucy was adamant that she wasn't happy with her body and wanted help in changing it. I like a challenge and Lucy was going to be just that.

Two days later Lucy visited me at my studio. My first impression of Lucy as she walked in was: 'WOW!' She is such a beautiful person and I couldn't help but wonder what she was seeing when she looked at herself in the mirror. We didn't waste any time and within five minutes of going through all the boring bits I had her on the treadmill for a quick warm-up and that's when we started to chat and I got to know her a bit better. I'm a firm believer in being connected to my clients because it's important to figure out where they are in their life, their beliefs, their fears, their loves and their hates. Straight away Lucy told me she hated the gym because she felt lost in there, never knowing what to do, self conscious of other people watching but most of all she found the experience boring.

I knew immediately that High-Intensity Interval Training (HIIT) was going to be the way to go for Lucy. It's fast, hard and it's easy to mix up each session, which is ideal for someone who is easily bored. Plus, it delivers the quick results she was looking for. The hardest challenge for me was to capture her attention and challenge her. Immediately she was 'hooked'. She wanted more and more and I had to put a programme together so that she had a focus of what to expect and when.

That first session consisted of 30 minutes of interval training, mixing cardio and resistance exercises and working all of her body parts.

Her focus was her bum and cellulite. She had seen pictures in the papers and magazines of herself on holiday and decided that she needed to get fit. Lucy thought that by exercise alone she'd be able to achieve her dream body but she needed to take into

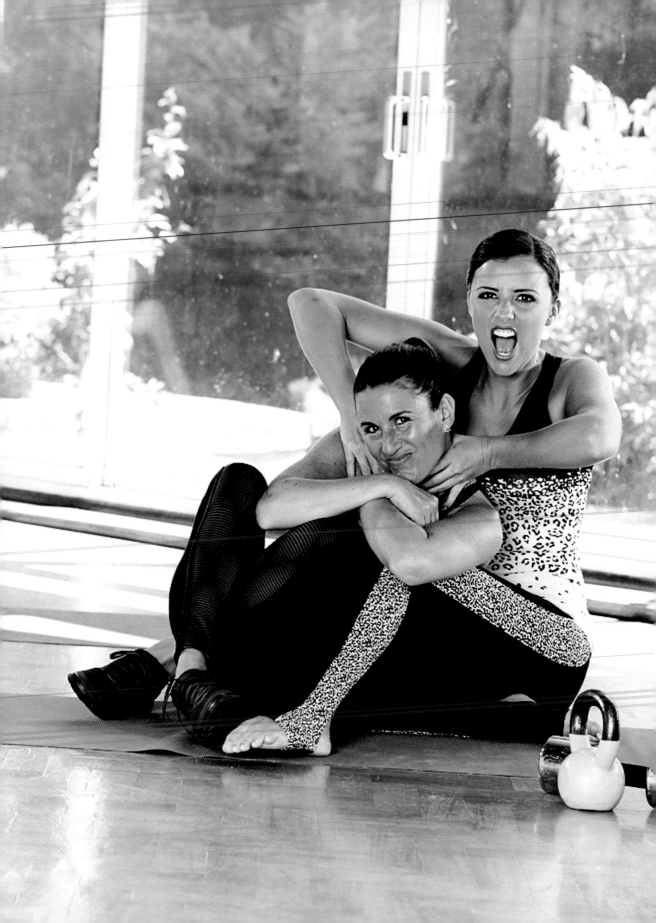

account all the other things making her feel lethargic and low. She needed to pay much more attention to her diet. Lucy never ate breakfast. Her lunch was either a salad or a sandwich and dinner was nearly always pasta – a recipe for disaster and a sure way to gain cellulite.

As you'll already know from reading the chapter on nutrition, cellulite is basically fatty deposits which sit under the surface of the skin and can look like little dimples. You can get rid of it easily enough, but it does take work and effort and, of course, eating the right foods.

I always tell my clients to change one thing at a time otherwise they find it overwhelming and can give up before they start. So, aside from the training, Lucy started to eat breakfast. A breakthrough. The saying 'fat people don't eat breakfast' is true.

Lucy began training three times a week for 30 minutes. My sessions are all 30 minutes long simply because I believe that exercise should be part of your day. If you are majorly over-ambitious it becomes impossible. Most people have busy lives that they have to fit exercise around. If it's too difficult then it's the first thing that goes. Mentally, 30 minutes of exercise works too because your brain can see the end

of half an hour. It doesn't sound so bad and your brain has already allowed you to think you can do it, which is a huge shift forwards.

But, in those 30 minutes you need to work harder than you have ever worked. I pushed Lucy through her comfort zone, working all of her body and by the end she would leave the sessions feeling positive, refreshed and ready to attack the world. It's really important to be in the right place mentally and while Lucy was working out I would talk to her and we would get closer and closer. At times it felt like I was more of a life coach than a fitness coach but it was incredibly rewarding. There were some days when Lucy would turn up feeling very down – particularly after her split with Mario – but by the end of the session she would be back to her positive self. She started to get her self-worth back and that was so important.

After the first week of training with Lucy I realised that she was a very determined person and loved a challenge, so our training sessions were increased to an hour session every other day. Her diet was significantly better and she was gradually cutting out as much sugar as possible (in Lucy's case that was the cocktails) and she was trading

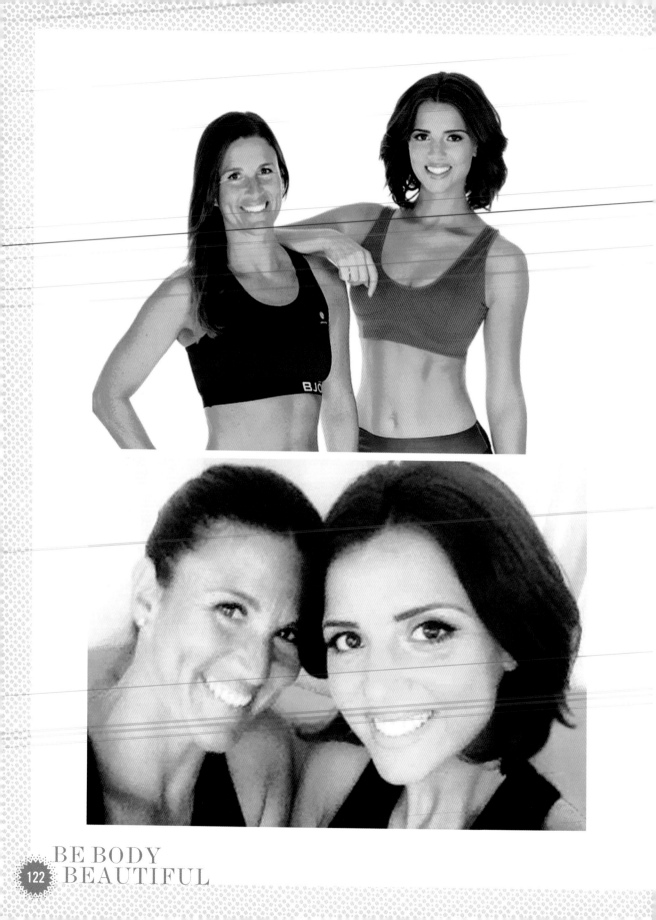

BE BODY
BEAUTIFUL

some of her beloved refined carbs like bread and pasta for quinoa, which she found she really liked.

Within four weeks she was seeing the changes. Her body 'leaned out' and was gaining muscle definition and, best of all, she was loving it. Her confidence was boosted as much as her energy levels and the better she looked the more attention she got.

But there was a setback. Part way through our initial training programme Lucy began filming for *TOWIE* again, and it was then that I started to notice changes in her. She became quiet and withdrawn and it was obvious that she was very stressed out. I wanted to help but it was hard because Lucy doesn't like to show any weakness or flaw. But I didn't give up, I dug a bit deeper, which is when she broke down and let it all out. *TOWIE* was beginning to stress her out a lot and the emphasis on the drama in her relationship with Mario was getting to her. She learned to lean on the training sessions as her way of getting away from it all.

However, her confidence started to wane and as things got worse in her personal life the strong Lucy was losing her spark again. I was determined not to let that happen, not to let her slip too far backwards. I had to build up her confidence by showing her she was

more capable than she believed, throwing more and more challenging exercise sessions at her. It was at about that time that the media picked up on the fact that she was getting too skinny. Her appetite was down because she was unhappy but what she was eating was healthy. Lucy is one of those people who loses weight with stress. Some people gain weight because of stress and comfort eating and some people are the opposite. Lucy is the second type. It was very clear that Lucy needed to change what made her unhappy in her life – and she did. She had the strength to move on from a toxic relationship and for the first time she bought a house – a place she could call her own and where there were no memories.

It wasn't an easy time but Lucy is incredibly strong when she wants to be and she threw herself into exercise and the things that made her feel good about herself … Her sheer determination and strength of character meant that instead of breaking down she made a bad situation turn around. Before long her body was the envy of her Twitter followers and they were asking us to post pictures of whole workouts online. That got us thinking: there was a business to be had …

Back to the story of the business. It gave me a new focus and another challenge. I am someone who needs challenging and this was something that I could really get my teeth stuck into. It's amazing being able to start a business that you are so passionate about. I can't imagine going back to a 'normal' job now or working behind a desk – that would be so weird. If I had to, of course I would, I just feel so lucky to be in the position I am. Fortunately, the business is doing amazingly well and we are getting more and more subscribers.

The aim of this business was to be different and to try and provide something completely unique for people wanting to get fit. There was obviously a gap in the market because it's what people were asking us for and in a way we were being led by them. The whole idea of making a fitness DVD feels a bit cheesy these days because everyone is doing them and when you see someone lose weight and then put it on again I think it dents the credibility of the workouts. I decided quite quickly that that wasn't for me. I wanted to start something that was fresh and new, something that I can update whenever I want to. It's far more immediate what we are doing. I also think that fitness DVDs can be quite boring for people and as someone who is easily bored I don't want to start boring other people with some mundane ninety-minute DVD workout bragging about how much you can lose in a ridiculously short length of time. It's been done by a lot of celebrities already and it just wasn't for me. On the whole those are quick fixes. Of course, there are exceptions to the rule, like Davina's DVDs, but I wanted to create a platform for long-term healthy living, not losing weight quickly to then pile it back on.

Primarily, I wanted to help young women. I wanted to make them enjoy exercise just like I do or, if they are coming to it later in life, to learn to enjoy it. Cecilia's husband, Frank, has the business head and agreed with us that the interest across social media could potentially become a new business. It was already being done in the US but in the UK there was nothing like what we wanted to do or nearly as big as we planned for our business to be. Together we agreed that

BE BODY
BEAUTIFUL

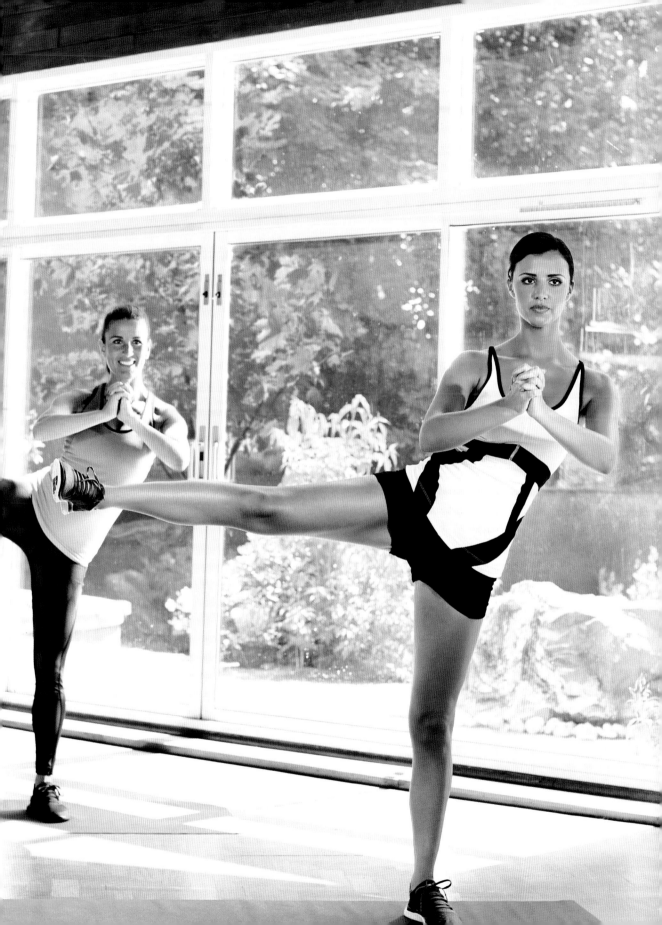

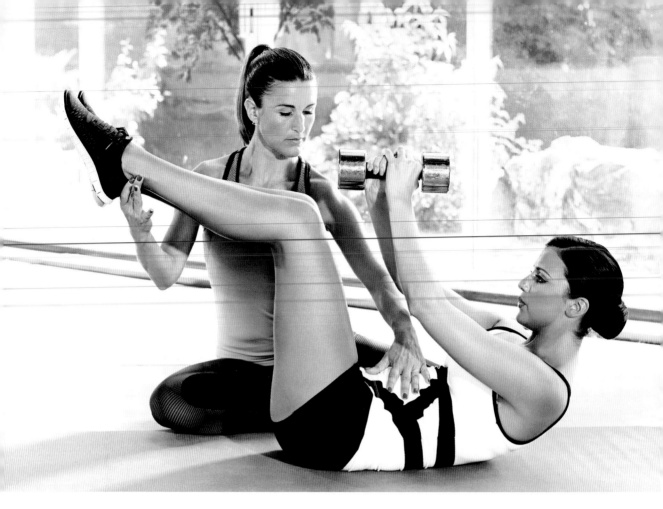

whatever we did should be an online platform for fitness and health that could grow and adapt.

Over the next few months we somehow managed to film nearly 300 different workouts. This sounds really weird, because I was filming for *TOWIE* and I should have been used to being in front of the camera, but I started to feel really self-conscious and almost got a bit camera shy. I found it really hard to talk directly to the camera rather than the camera just being around me as it was on *TOWIE*. I felt sort of embarrassed in a way but I needed to get over it if the website was going to work. It helped me to see that the most popular videos were the ones where Cecilia and I were interacting or having fun together and giggling. Basically, having a bit of banter between us. Once I knew people liked what we were doing I got a bit more

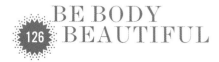

BE BODY BEAUTIFUL

confident and gradually I started to relax in front of the camera. That was until I had to say actual pieces to camera. I had to literally stand there and talk directly to the camera as if I was talking to the person wanting to do the workout. It was so weird and I felt more self-conscious than ever. God knows how many times I had to re-record my pieces. I'd usually screw up my lines or start laughing or want to sneeze. It's quite funny looking back now but at the time I got so frustrated with myself. I hate not being able to do something and the more I tried the worse it seemed to get. I don't suppose the person filming me thought it was very funny after take twenty-eight either! In a way I suppose this helped me with *Tumble* a bit because I had to do lots of pieces to camera and if I'd messed those up too many times I don't think the BBC would have been very happy with me! I'd have gone through about a hundred videotapes!

Alongside making the videos we were building the website (called Resultswithlucy.com) to put the videos on. It was quite scary because I had no idea where to start with building a website. I was reliant on the people around me to make the product work. I provided the materials to go on it and the ideas, but that was about as much as I could do. My dad has always – actually he still does – done so many things for me. Dad is a businessman, he's sharp and dynamic. He deals with the accountant or if I need to get something done he will sort it out for me so I'd never had to properly stand on my own two feet. If I need anything Dad is there but I wanted to make him proud and show him what I could do. I was still a bit reliant on him helping me, though! I have no idea how to do accounting or bookkeeping or anything like that. I'm a nightmare. I don't even own a laptop! But I do work extremely hard, have creative ideas and run with them, and I never give up on anything.

The website was an instant success. I still can't believe how mad everyone went for it, from the moment we launched it. I remember the day, though, because it was just so amazing.

 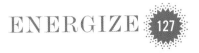

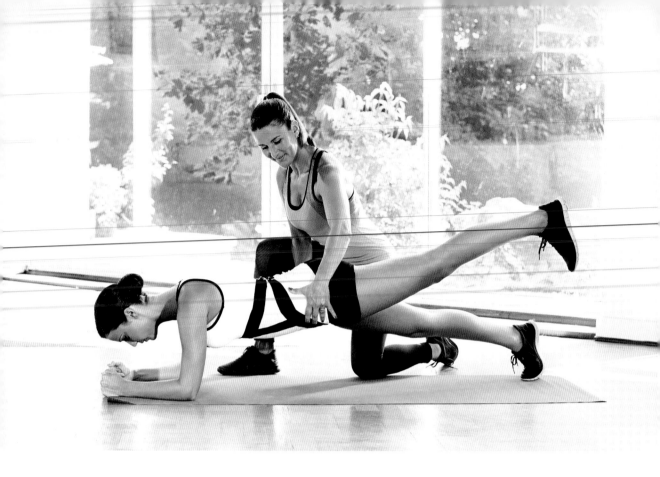

It was 24 June 2013 and by that point we had been tweeting workouts for over a month and I was just about to announce to my followers the launch of the website. Cecilia, Frank and I all sat in a room in front of a laptop which showed us a graph with live figures for how many people were visiting the site. As I sent the tweet, the graph went from zero to two thousand in just under a minute. It was nuts. We were like kids in a playground just jumping up and down with joy. All the hard work had paid off and it felt like such an amazing achievement. I just wanted to go out and celebrate with a few cocktails!

Life became busy then because not only did I have the website – which was going amazingly – but I also had my two boutiques, which do very well, and I didn't want to take my focus off any of the projects. It was hard as there was so much going on, plus I was still filming *TOWIE*. My agent, Scarlett (who is like a big sister to me and has

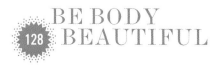

been with me through absolutely everything), and I were travelling all over, shooting campaigns abroad and at home and I was having the time of my life. Scarlett once gave me some advice – well, she's given me lots throughout the years, ha ha! – but this always sticks in my mind. She said that people who find fame quickly, and are plastered over every magazine for all the wrong reasons, rarely last long and if they do it's because their lives are a car crash. She knew I wasn't like that and that to have longevity in the media industry you have to be patient and hardworking and want people to aspire to be like you for all the right reasons. And then the rest will fall into place.

Patience is definitely a virtue and if I'm going to do something I like to do it properly. I can't stand the idea of doing something half-heartedly, it's not the way I'm made. Add my training to all that and you can see I was pretty damn busy! I was still training every other day. If I'm going to be an advocate for fitness routines I don't want people looking at me and seeing cellulite on me or a body they wouldn't like to have. That's not exactly inspirational for them so I worked really hard to stay fit and cellulite free!

My diet was being looked after by Emma and it was around then that she came on board with the business too. She has been amazing because exercise and nutrition go hand in hand. I wouldn't have been able to do *Tumble* if I hadn't upped my food intake. I love food so that didn't bother me, but you have to recognize that if you are going to train more you need to eat more too or your body won't handle it.

The EatWell with Lucy diet was personalized for me so that it would suit my lifestyle, help specifically with cellulite but also energy levels, bloating and stress. It was life-changing for me and really propped me up while I was so busy. The website continues to go from strength to strength and we have created a real community of people who are encouraging one another too, which is brilliant.

I try to think of new ideas all the time to keep the website fresh and now we don't just offer exercise routine videos but we also offer Pilates, yoga, combat, circuits, stretching and relaxing videos (which teach you how to completely switch off after a busy day). The variety

 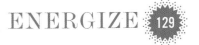

of options we now have to offer has really kept our audience growing and coming back for more, which is what I dreamed of happening. The worst thing I could do at this point is to sit back, just think it's working fine and not come up with new, fresh ideas that can move the business on. That's the beauty of a website – anything can be changed, at any time.

Exercise is a bit of an enigma for some people. They are scared of doing it. Maybe it's the fear of failure or of not getting the results or simply because, like me, the idea of going to a gym or boot camp fills them with complete dread. The thing is I was that person but I've got over it and if I can then you can too – but you have to want to. It's no good talking about it or thinking about it, you need to get the ball rolling and get out there and make the change. Running is a cheap way of getting fit but I know a lot of people feel very self-conscious about it. But how often do you look and judge someone jogging along the road? You don't, and the same goes for other people looking at you. People are in their own worlds and aren't staring at you. In truth they are probably thinking, 'I need to get fit like them.' You need to get things into perspective and not use these thoughts as a reason not to get on with it. Even if it's just for ten minutes a day, something is better than nothing and it will boost your confidence to do more.

Don't drag your heels any more. Wake up tomorrow and make the change. Go for a walk, a short run or do a few exercises at home like some squats, some lunges and a couple of press-ups. Even 10 minutes a day will start to change you. Once you have started you will want more because you will feel good about achieving something.

Your body will ache a little but there's no gain without a bit of pain and if you are aching then you know that it's working and doing something. You will feel satisfied and proud of yourself for getting moving and that boosts self-esteem, confidence, everything. It's a real tonic.

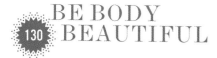

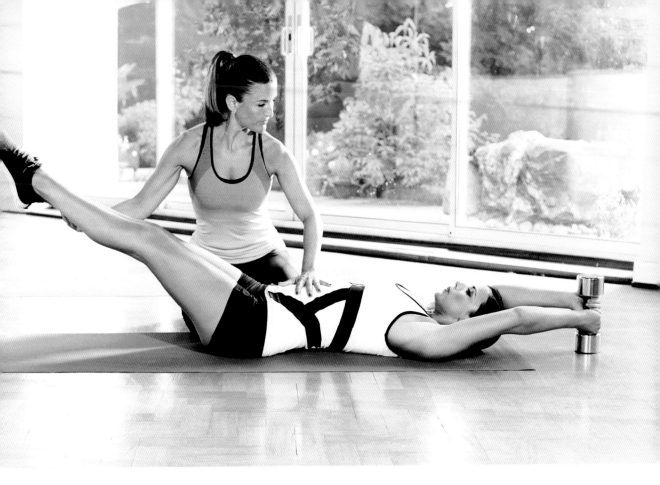

Slowly build up your exercise each day. Mix it up a bit and vary your workout so you don't get bored. Don't be shy, you will find something that you love and stick to for a while, but don't always do the same routine. Changing it up regularly, I find, is the key to success. Equally some people like going for a run while others prefer the gym and others prefer classes. As you know I hate the gym but I do love going to classes. Having people around me pushing themselves and a teacher at the front encouraging us, are really helpful to me. Find what you enjoy because you are much more likely to stick with exercise if you enjoy it.

One of my favourite quotes is: 'Fitness is not a destination, it's a lifestyle.' Fitness has to be part of our lives, just like brushing our teeth. Don't fall into the trap of being one of these people who only gets fit before going on holiday or a party or a wedding. It's a lifestyle

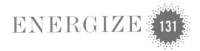

ENERGIZE 131

change and yo-yoing like that is hard work and not good for your body because it never knows where it stands.

I've already mentioned my bootycamps and they are kind of like a weekend class for people, where they often cleanse their minds as well as their bodies.

I think they are popular because, unlike other boot camps, they don't beat you down and make you feel vulnerable and miserable. I am planning a load more. The first camp I ran was on 31 January 2014 and it was spread over three days. I couldn't believe how many people signed up for it and 180 ladies attended. It was incredible. Having 180 women training in one place – the energy was unreal. We began the day all together with a group workout, which is really feel-good. I can't even explain the feeling of training so many people! And it really encourages people to keep going when everyone does it together. Because the camp lasted for a few days, the girls start to make little friendship/support groups and I'm sure a lot of them have stayed in touch afterwards, which can only help encourage them to continue working out. It's a journey, but it's a lifetime journey so you might as well enjoy it!

Here are a couple of the letters that I received after that first bootycamp. They mean so much to me and are an inspiration to anyone wanting to lose that weight or make that change to their lives.

'FITNESS IS A LIFETIME JOURNEY SO YOU MIGHT AS WELL ENJOY IT!'

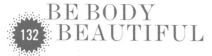

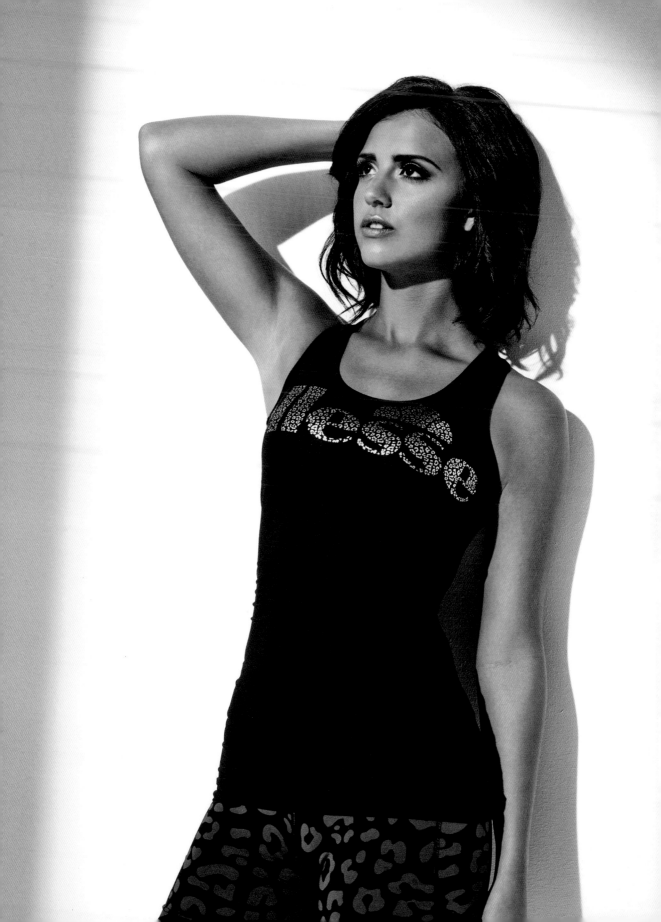

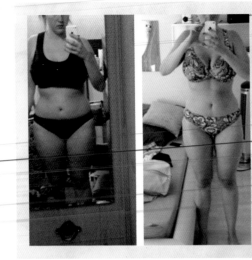

CLAIRE:
'I AM SO MUCH HAPPIER,
AND INTEND FOR THIS
PLAN TO BE A PART OF
MY LIFE FOR EVER.'

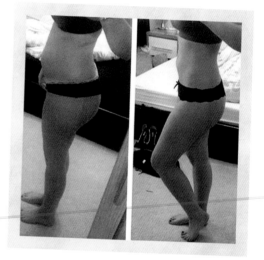

LAURA BURNS:
'I AM SO HAPPY THAT I
JOINED RESULTS WITH LUCY.
IT HAS COMPLETELY
CHANGED MY LIFE.'

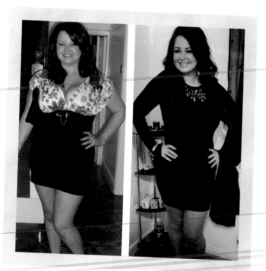

KATIE WALKER:
'I FEEL SO MUCH MORE CONFIDENT,
AND NOW I AM SEEING A DIFFERENCE.
I FINALLY FEEL LIKE I HAVE CONQUERED
THE BATTLE WITH MY WEIGHT.'

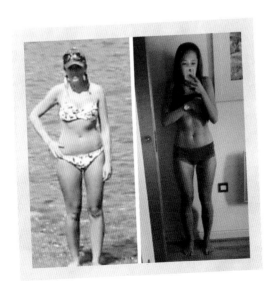

JESSIE HYNES:
'I FEEL MUCH LIGHTER,
SLIMMER, MORE DEFINED
AND, MOST IMPORTANTLY,
MUCH FITTER IN MYSELF.
I FEEL DETERMINED TO
CONTINUE WITH THE VALUES
THAT THE PROGRAMME
HAS TAUGHT ME! WOULD
100% RECOMMEND IT.'

LOUISE O'TOOLE:
'MY MUSCLES HAVE MORE
DEFINITION, MY HAIR
AND SKIN ARE BETTER,
I'M FITTER AND HEALTHIER
AND I FEEL SO MUCH
HAPPIER. IT'S ADDICTIVE!
I FEEL AMAZING.'

I have been incredibly fortunate to be able to make a living out of something I love and have such passion for, and I'm eternally grateful for that. The fact that I got to be part of *Tumble* last year was amazing too. It took a lot of hard work but it made me feel so good about myself and I am really proud that I managed not to make a fool of myself and that I sustained that level of training. If I hadn't been as fit as I was then my body never could have done it, that's for sure. I was also in a good place mentally. Although I was terrified on the first night, I knew that I had got myself into the best possible shape to be able to compete. I had never done gymnastics before and that was nerve-wracking because it was outside my comfort zone for a start. I needed to prepare as much as I could. As soon as I was signed up I started to follow a training plan that would help me with my upper body strength and flexibility.

Our movement therapist at Results with Lucy, Liam Willis, helped me with my flexibility by using three-dimensional movement and his in-depth knowledge of biomechanics in my training. Humans are designed to move in three dimensions: forwards/backwards and sideways. Rarely in real life do any of us do things in a robotic, one- or two-dimensional way. Just try picking up a cup of coffee from the table and you'll see how your hand moves backwards towards your body, sideways towards your mouth, and perfectly to your lips with a final twist.

You can apply that same breakdown to nearly every large movement we make. Working out this way ensures that you build muscles that are long, lean and flexible. It also makes you less prone to injury because you are so much more flexible.

You can't underestimate how important it is that exercise mirrors our natural movements, whether that's lifting, turning, reaching or stooping. This is something that I have always put at the heart of our fitness programmes. Work with your body not against it. The last thing you want is an injury. Something I often got in *Tumble*!

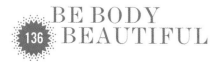

While I was on *Tumble* I carried on with high-intensity interval training to build my fitness level, and I did a lot more bodyweight exercises to build my strength. I had to familiarize myself as much as possible with all the different gymnastics equipment, like the vault and the beam, which were completely foreign to me. I could have been stupidly scared but I wanted to embrace it and try something new that would push me right out of my comfort zone. *Tumble* definitely did that. It was a brilliant experience and one I will never forget – not least for the new bum I got!

Have I inspired you enough to put on your trainers and get going? I hope so. I've put together some sample workouts, so there's no excuse! N.B. If you're going to get moving right now, make sure you warm up and warm down and drink plenty of water. And for those of you wanting to follow my six-week exercise plan, which will guarantee you a new body shape, weight, dress size and outlook on life, keep reading. It's all coming up soon (pages 225–41).

Remember. You CAN do it. Fact.

 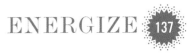

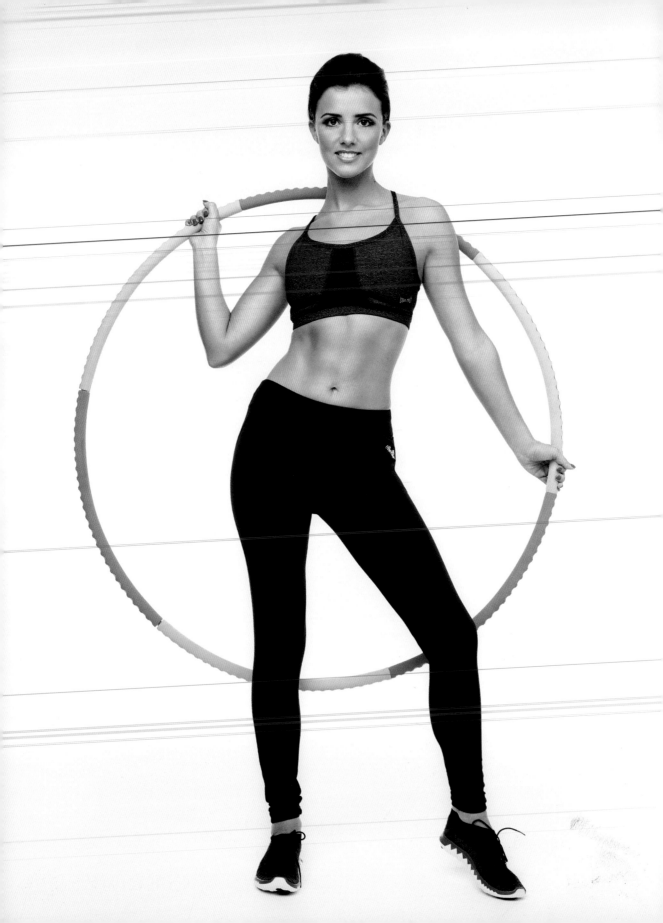

MY 'EXERCISE AT HOME' ROUTINE

1 Alternate Lunges
Fitness focus: quads (the fronts of your thighs)

Standing with feet together,
Hands on hips,
Take a large step forwards with your right leg.
Bend both knees so you lower yourself to the ground.
Your back knee should not quite touch the floor.
Keep your chest up and shoulders back.
From here return to your start position and repeat on
your other leg.
Repeat 30 times.

2 Squat into Jumping Jacks
Fitness focus: quads, calves, cardio (cardiovascular
exercise raises your heart rate and in turn makes your
metabolism move faster)

Standing with feet together,
Squat down.
Keep your knees and feet together,
Back nice and straight,
Chest up,
Hands clasped in front of you at chest height.
From here jump up, spreading your legs.
Land with your feet about 1½ times shoulder width apart.

 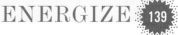

At the same time raise your arms straight out to the side.
Keep your belly button pulled in,
Head up.
Jump back to the start position.
Repeat 15 times.

3 Press-ups
Fitness focus: chest (the muscle above your boobs –
chest exercises are good for lifting your boobs) and triceps
(these are your bingo wings!)

Place your hands 1½ times shoulder width apart,
Fingers pointing forwards,
Knees and feet together, knees on the floor.
Keeping your hips up, make as straight a line as possible
from hips to shoulders.
Keep your belly button pulled in.
Breathe in as you bend your elbows, flaring them out to
the side.
Do not allow your head to sag, keep your neck in line with
your spine.
As you lower yourself down try to make a triangle pattern
with your hands and forehead.
You should not finish with your head in line with your hands.
With your back nice and straight squeeze your chest and the
backs of your arms.
Breathe out as you return to your start position.
Repeat 10 times.

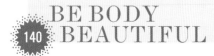

4 Crunches
Fitness focus: abs (between your belly button and your boobs)

Lying on your back,
Knees bent,
Feet flat,
Hands by your temples,
Elbows out.
Squeeze your abs and lift your upper back off the floor.
Breathe out as you lift, pulling your belly button down.
Keep a gap between your chin and your chest.
Breathe in as you return to the floor.
Repeat 15 times.

5 Legs-up Crunch
Fitness focus: abs

Lying on your back,
Lift your feet into the air,
Legs straight,
Belly button pulled in.
Squeeze your abs and lift your upper back off the floor.
Try to touch your toes with your fingers.
Breathe out as you lift, pulling your belly button down.
Keep a gap between your chin and your chest.
Breathe in as you return to the floor.
Repeat 10 times.

6 Plank
Fitness focus: abs, shoulders, back

Lying face down, place your elbows directly under your shoulders.
Keep your feet and knees together with the weight on your toes.
Lift your hips in line with your shoulders creating a tabletop back.
(You should be able to rest your favourite drink without
spilling a drop!)
Keep your belly button pulled in tightly, making your waist
as small as possible.
Don't allow your head to drop down. Make sure it is in alignment
with your spine.
**Hold the plank position for 5 to 10 seconds at a time for a total
of 1 minute.**

You will feel fitter each time you perform this routine. Therefore,
as you improve, increase the reps and hold the plank for longer.
Aim to complete this workout five days each week, with two
non-consecutive rest days.

'YOU WILL FEEL FITTER
EVERYTIME YOU PERFORM THIS ROUTINE.
TRUST ME,
REGULAR EXERCISE WILL
CHANGE YOUR LIFE.'

BE BODY
BEAUTIFUL

MY 'EXERCISE IN THE PARK' ROUTINE

1 Side Leap
Fitness Focus: inner thighs, quads, calves, glutes
(your butt cheeks)

Stand on a flat surface with your feet together.
Bend your knees and hop as far as you can to your right,
landing on the ball of your right foot.
Without returning your left foot to the ground, bend your
right knee and hop as far as you can to the left.
Work up to 20 hops on each side.

2 Park-bench Dip
Fitness Focus: triceps, shoulders, abs

Sit on a bench and place your hands on either side of your hips.
Slide your bum forwards, supporting yourself with your hands.
Bend your elbows, bringing your upper arms almost parallel
to the ground, then return to the starting position.
Complete 12 to 15 reps.
Tip: Keep your lower back close to the bench throughout
the exercise.

 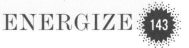

3 Park-bench Press-up
Fitness Focus: chest, biceps, triceps, shoulders, abs

Stand facing a bench and place your hands on the seat.
Walk your feet out behind you until your legs are fully
extended.
Bend your arms and lower your chest towards the bench,
Then push up.
Complete 12 reps.

Turn around and place your hands on the ground and your
feet on the bench.
Walk your hands forwards until they're aligned under
your shoulders,
Legs extended.
Lower your chest towards the ground,
Then push up.
Complete 8 reps.

As you get fitter, work up to 20 reps of each.

4 Side Shuffle
Fitness Focus: glutes, inner and outer thighs, quads

Stand with your feet hip distance apart,
Elbows bent, with your fists near your ribs.
Take three giant steps to your right, sliding your left foot
to meet the right each time.
Bend your knees and jump up, turning through 180 degrees
to face the opposite direction.
Repeat, shuffling to your left.
Continue alternating sides for 1 minute.

BE BODY
BEAUTIFUL

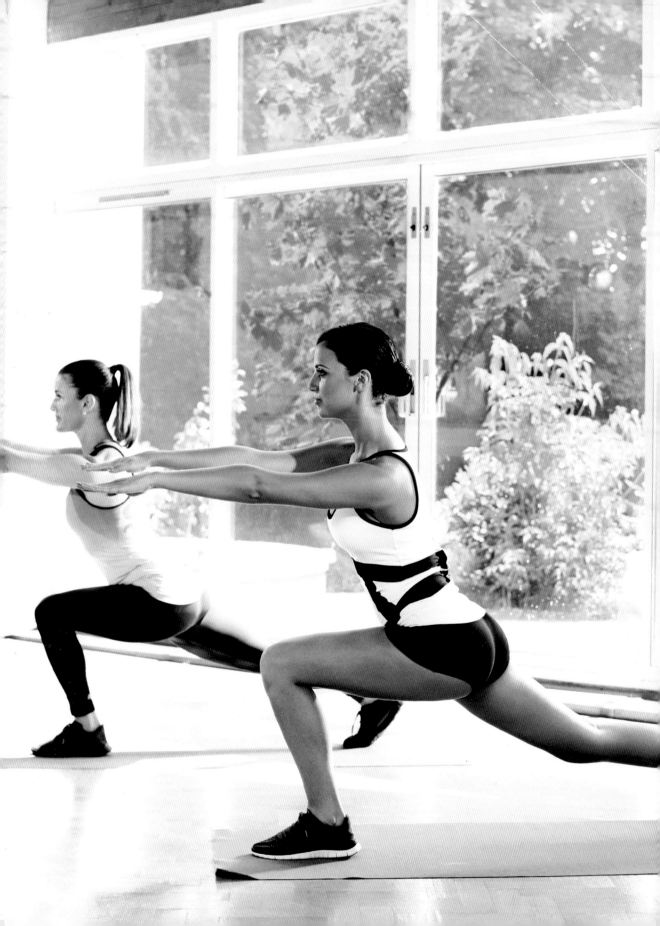

5 Side Step

Fitness Focus: abs, obliques (the muscles at the sides of your tummy – they accentuate your waistline and give you definition), glutes, upper back, shoulders

Stand with your right side facing a step, log or flat rock.
Hold your arms out to your sides at shoulder height.
Bend your elbows through ninety degrees, palms facing forwards.
Step up with your right foot,
Contract your abs,
While bringing your left knee and right elbow together in front of you.
(Emphasize bringing your knee up rather than your elbow down.)
Return to the starting position.
Complete 12 reps on each side.

6 Abdominal Hold

Fitness Focus: abs

Sit tall on the edge of a bench.
Place your hands on the edge with your fingers pointing towards your knees.
Tighten your abs and bring your toes 5–10cm off the floor.
Lift your bum off the bench.
Hold this position for as long as you can – aim for 5–10 seconds.
Lower yourself down and repeat.
Continue for 1 minute.

BE BODY
BEAUTIFUL

'THE ACCUMULATOR' WORKOUT

Already fit but want to push yourself a bit harder? The accumulator will help you tone up and feel great. This workout is for the intermediate/advanced level. It's called the accumulator because the routine uses the perfect combo of body weight and cardiovascular exercises to lose weight and gain muscle definition.

This workout consists of a number of exercises that you do for 30 seconds at a time. You will start with one exercise for 30 seconds and add another but you must always start from your first exercise. Got it? Here goes...

- Squat and kick up your legs alternately for 30 seconds. (exercise 1)
- Rest 10 seconds.
- Squat and kick for 30 seconds. (exercise 1)
- Sprint forwards, touch the floor, sprint backwards, touch the floor for 30 seconds. (exercise 2)
- Rest 10 seconds.
- Squat and kick for 30 seconds. (exercise 1)
- Sprint forwards and backwards for 30 seconds. (exercise 2)
- Get into a plank position on the floor and do the mountain climber movement (holding the plank bring one knee at a time to your chest and back) for 30 seconds. (exercise 3)
- Rest for 10 seconds.
- Squat and kick for 30 seconds. (exercise 1)
- Sprint forwards and backwards for 30 seconds. (exercise 2)
- Get into a plank position on the floor and do the mountain climber for 30 seconds. (exercise 3)
- Press-ups for 30 seconds. (exercise 4)
- Rest 10 seconds.

- ★ Start again from squat and kick for 30 seconds (exercises 1–4) and after your press-ups add:
- ★ Jumping squats for 30 seconds. (exercise 5)
- ★ Rest 10 seconds.
- ★ Start again from squat and kick for 30 seconds (exercises 1–5) and after your jumping squats add:
- ★ Alternate lunges for 30 seconds. (exercise 6)
- ★ Rest for 10 seconds.

How are you feeling? By now your legs should be burning and your heart rate pumping. As you get fitter, you can repeat the whole routine.

If you are after more muscle definition, just add weights. Squat and shoulder press (press the weights straight upwards) with dumbbells of 3–5kg instead of the squats and kicks. Hold the dumbbells when doing alternate lunges. Add an exercise like bicep curls for 30 seconds to the accumulator.

Bicep Curls

Standing nice and tall, holding one dumbbell in each hand, place your feet hip width apart. Make your tummy nice and tight, and slightly tilt your pelvis forwards so that you don't arch your back. Bring the dumbbells up towards your shoulders but keep your upper arms close to your body. Try to only move the arms and not swing forwards and backwards, so that only your biceps are working.

I hope you've enjoyed these tasters (there's still much more to come with the Six-week Plan – pages 225–41). For more of my exercise routines visit www.resultswithlucy.com.

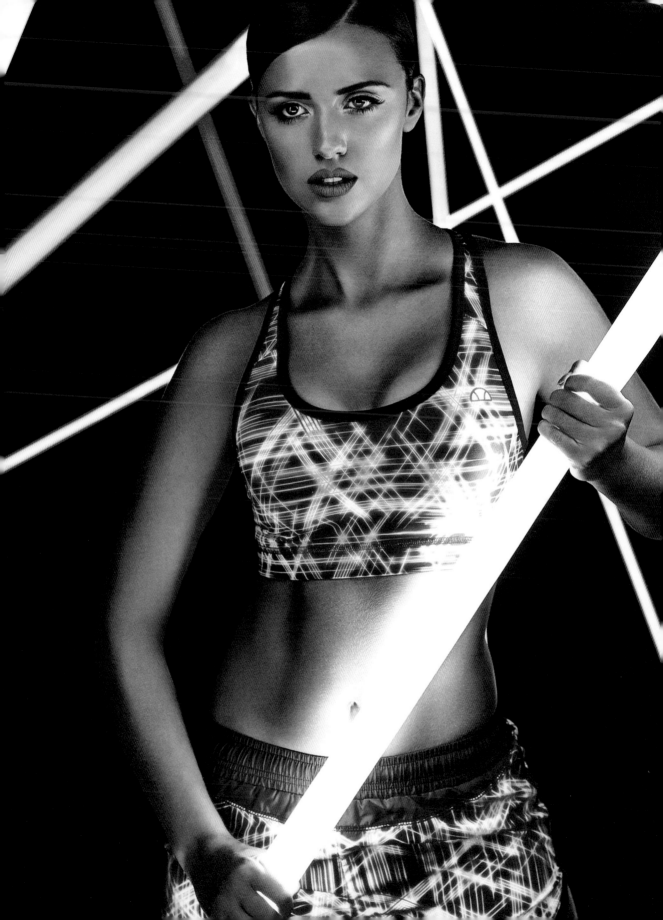

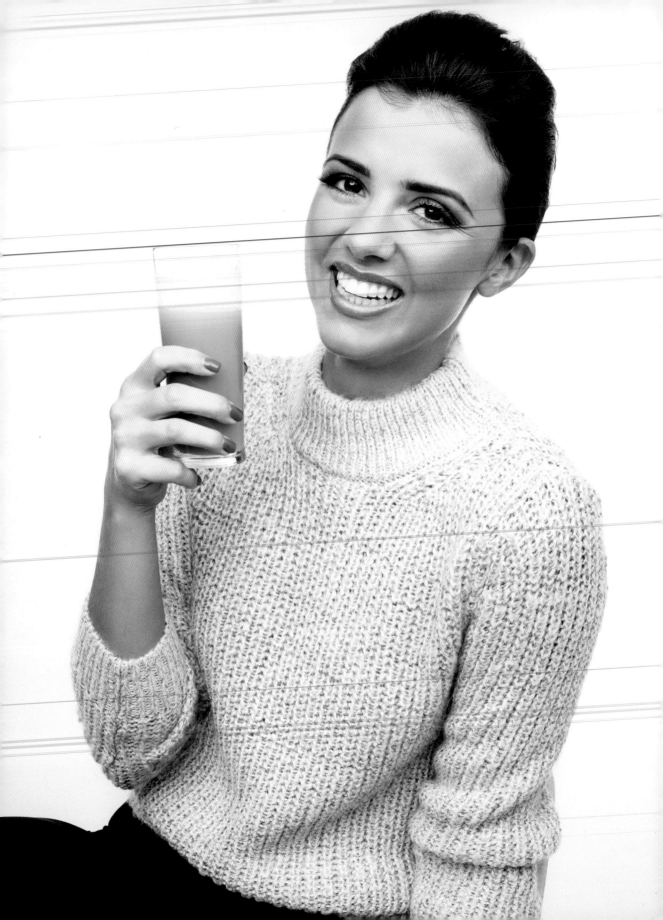

5
THE RECIPES

The food you eat has a huge impact on how you look and feel. Gillian McKeith was right all those years ago – you really are what you eat! Your diet can transform your mood, help you lose weight, sleep better and boost your energy levels. In this chapter I'll share some of my favourite recipes. Hope you love them as much as I do!

N.B. Use a cup measuring approximately 240ml for these recipes.

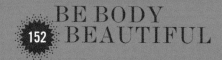

GREEN GODDESS SMOOTHIE

1 banana
a handful of baby spinach
    leaves
1 tsp spirulina powder
flesh of ½ a medium avocado
1 tsp natural honey
500ml water

SERVES 1
2–3 MINS TO MAKE

This delicious smoothie cleanses my body and
keeps toxins under control, which helps me to
balance my life and helps my body to recover
from the occasional night out!

>–●–<–>–●–<

Blend together and devour!

ALMOND MILK SMOOTHIE

2 cups organic almond milk
2 large frozen peeled
   bananas
2–3 fresh dates, pitted
   and diced
a dash of vanilla extract or
   ¼ tsp ground cinnamon

SERVES 1
2–3 MINS TO MAKE

Almond milk is a great alternative to cows
milk. It doesn't cause bloating and keeps
my tummy flat.

Combine all the ingredients together in
a high-speed blender.

MALIBU BEACH SMOOTHIE

1 banana
½ cup fresh pineapple
   chunks
½ cup coconut milk
½ cup coconut water

SERVES 1
2–3 MINS TO MAKE

I love being on holiday and this reminds me of
being on a beach. It's healthy and pineapple is
great for digestion and boosting metabolism.

Combine all the ingredients together in
a high-speed blender.

ALMOND & DATE SMOOTHIE

5 dates, pitted and chopped
1 tbsp raw almond butter
120ml almond milk
120ml water
1 tsp natural honey
1 banana

SERVES 1
2–3 MINS TO MAKE

Dates are naturally sweet, so when I am looking
for something to kick the sugar craving, I have
an almond and date smoothie.

Blend all the ingredients together in
a high-speed blender.

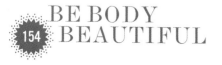

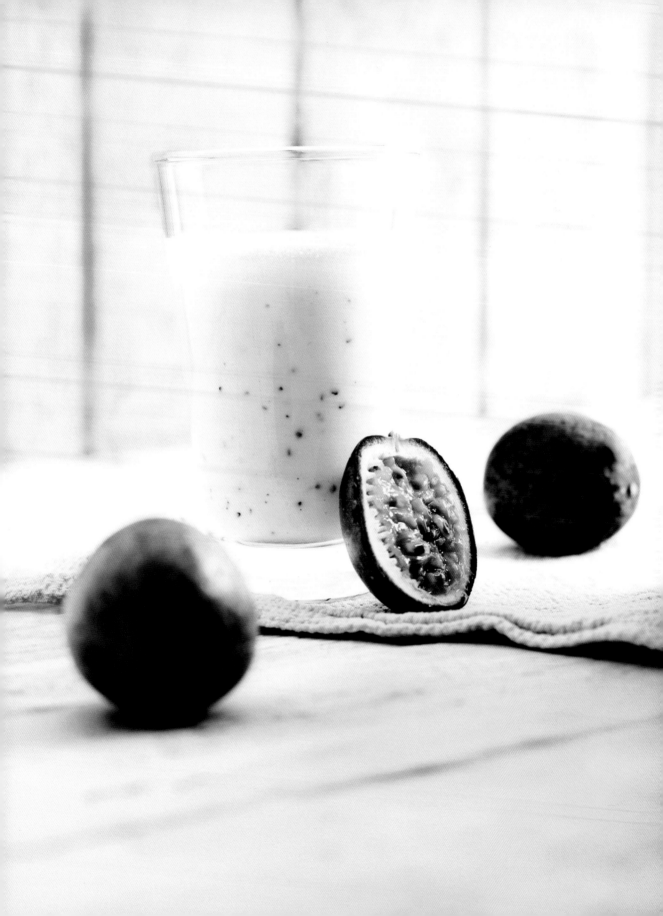

BANANA BERRY SMOOTHIE

1 banana
1 cup fresh or frozen
   strawberries or
   mixed berries
1 tsp natural honey
½ cup filtered water

SERVES 1
2–3 MINS TO MAKE

I love this smoothie. I have bananas at the start the day for energy, and the berries are antioxidants – brilliant beauty food.

Combine all the ingredients together in a high-speed blender.

CLEAN & CLEAR SMOOTHIE

a handful of spinach leaves
a handful of kale,
   roughly chopped
1 cup broccoli florets
1 large or 2 small bananas
½ cup fresh pineapple
optional: 1 tsp squeezy
   organic honey
   (if needed to sweeten)
300ml water

SERVES 1
2–3 MINS TO MAKE

This is another beauty food. It is high in antioxidants and is great for cleansing and anti-ageing.

Combine all the ingredients in a high-speed blender, then drink.

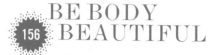

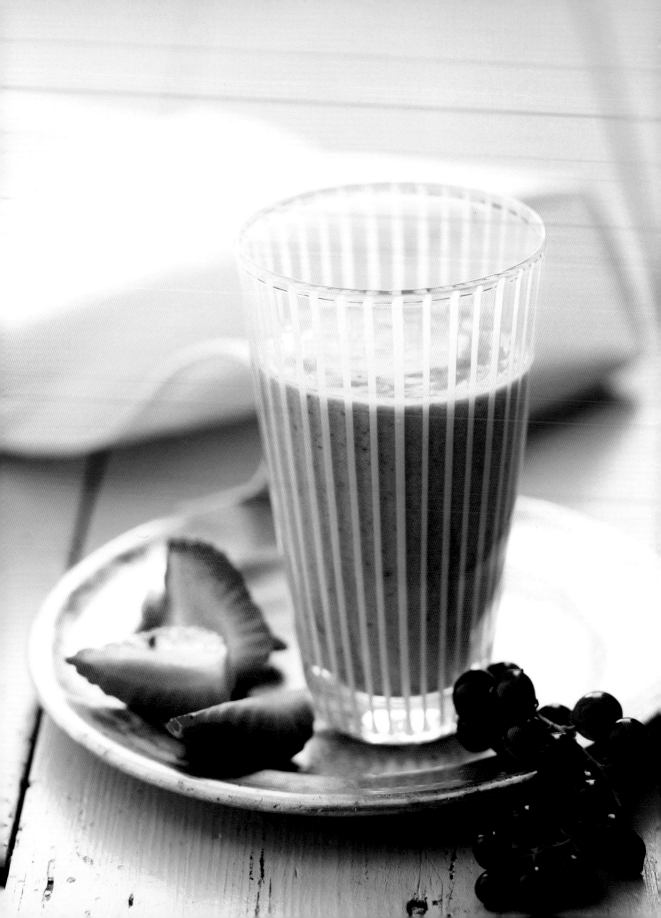

ANTIOXIDANT BLEND

just-boiled water
2 organic green tea bags
1 cup blueberries
1 cup raspberries
2 tsp honey

SERVES 1
4–5 MINS TO MAKE, PLUS
CHILLING AND OVERNIGHT
SOAKING TIME

Another beauty food that has a huge number of health benefits. It contains green tea which is an anti-cancer agent.

Pour the boiled water over the green tea bags in a mug and leave to stand for an hour to cool. Then cover the mug with cling film and place it in the fridge overnight. In the morning, remove the tea bags and blend the cold green tea, berries and honey in a blender, then enjoy!

MAGIC MACA SMOOTHIE

1 tbsp maca powder
2–3 tbsp cocoa powder
1 cup almond milk
1–1½ cups filtered water
3 fresh dates, pitted
flesh of 1 small avocado
optional: 1 tsp pure
    vanilla extract

SERVES 1
2–3 MINS TO MAKE

Maca is great for hormone balance and perfect taken in the last ten days of your menstrual cycle.

Blend all the ingredients together and enjoy.

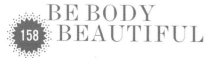

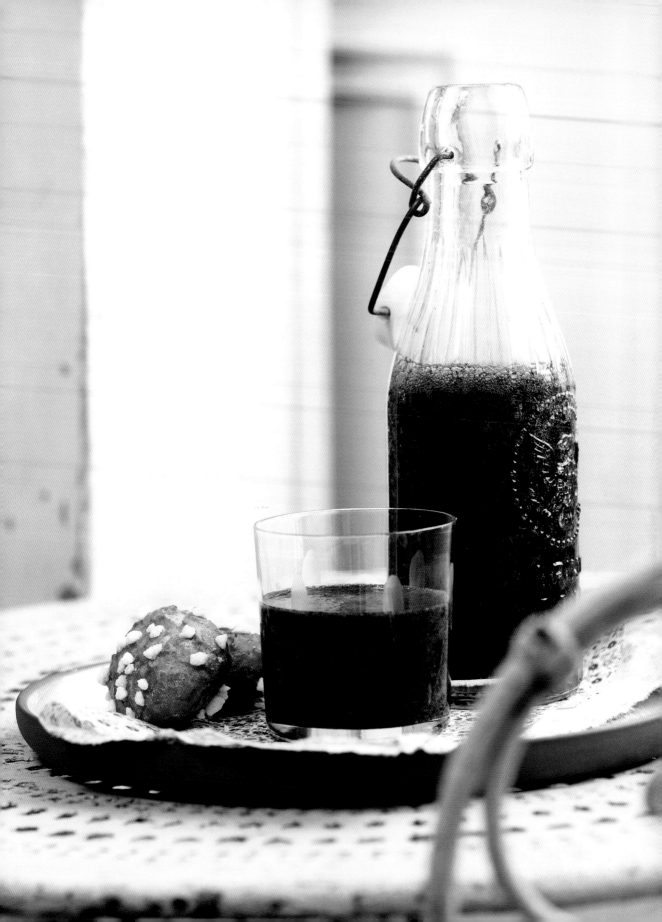

NATURAL PORRIDGE

1 cup porridge oats (ideally organic oats, but definitely not the instant stuff!)

1½–2 cups water

whatever toppings you choose, such as chopped fresh apple and a sprinkling of ground cinnamon, banana slices and a little desiccated coconut or mixed berries and a drizzle of honey

SERVES 1
10 MINS TO MAKE

TIP
Ideally steel-cut oats are the best, then organic oats or finally good-quality standard porridge oats. Just look at the ingredients list on the packet, which should only say 100% oats!

TIP
You may need to add a bit more water if the oats soak it all up too quickly. The best way to see if they are done is to have a taste!

I like nothing better on a cold wintry morning than to curl up on my sofa with a big bowl of porridge. It's perfect comfort food and keeps hunger locked up till lunch! Try my recipe below for the perfect start to the day.

Put the oats into a medium saucepan and add enough water to just cover the top of the oats. Bring it to a boil then turn down to a simmer, stirring regularly. The porridge will be ready when the oats have soaked up all the water but the mixture still has a runny texture. The cooking time will partly depend on what 'cut' or grade of oats you've used. Serve in bowls, with your chosen toppings.

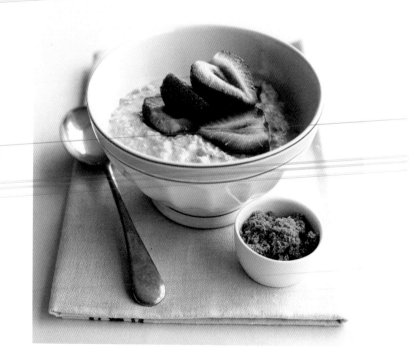

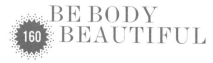

BE BODY
BEAUTIFUL

PURPLE PORRIDGE

2 tbsp medium or fine
    oatmeal or porridge oats
1 tbsp desiccated coconut
a pinch of salt
freshly boiled water
1 large tsp manuka honey
½ cup frozen blueberries
1 tbsp ground flaxseed
    mix (Linwoods brand
    or similar)
optional toppings: almond
    or oat milk, sliced banana,
    coco nibs

SERVES 1
5 MINS TO MAKE

This is basically porridge, but with added
nutrients, which makes it even better for
you than normal porridge!

Place all the dry ingredients except the ground
flaxseed in a small saucepan and cover with boiling
water. Bring up to a low heat, stirring continuously
so it doesn't stick, until the mixture starts to thicken.
Add more water if needed to keep a good consistency.
Stir in the honey and blueberries, until the porridge
turns purple from the blueberries. Just before
serving, add the flaxseed mix and add a little more
water again, if needed. Serve with almond milk,
coco nibs and slices of fresh banana, as you like.

COCONUT BERRY SALAD

½ cup fresh or frozen
    raspberries (if using
    frozen, defrost first)
1 tsp natural honey
2 pieces of organic dark
    chocolate (minimum
    70% cocoa solids)
1 tbsp desiccated coconut

*Equipment: you will
need a mini grater
(for the chocolate).*

SERVES 1
2–3 MINS TO MAKE

Coconut is full of healthy fats that keep your
skin, hair and nails looking good, plus the berries
provide an injection of antioxidants for your skin.
An all-round winner!

Place the raspberries in a bowl. Swirl the honey over
the berries and stir to coat. Grate the chocolate on top
and then sprinkle on the coconut, to form a thick
dusting that covers the berries.

 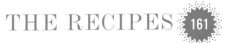

BREAKFAST 'ROUGHIE'

¼ cup ground flaxseed
¼ cup rye flakes or
    porridge oats
1 tbsp desiccated coconut
1 banana
1 cup frozen berries (any
    kind of berries will do)
¾ cup almond or rice milk
optional: ¼ cup filtered
    water (for a thinner
    consistency)
2 tsp natural honey

SERVES 1
2–3 MINS TO MAKE

This is a very simple, quick and easy complete breakfast in a drink!

⊃·⊛·○·⊃·⊛·○

Put the flaxseed, rye or oats, coconut and fruit together in the jug of a high-speed blender. Then add the milk, water (if using) and, finally, the honey. Blend together to make a rough breakfast drink.

SAVOURY SCRAMBLE

1 tsp coconut oil
2 eggs, beaten
a handful of chopped
    fresh parsley
1 spring onion, thinly sliced
1 medium or 6 cherry
    tomatoes, sliced and diced
salt and pepper, to season
3 handfuls of baby spinach
    leaves
optional: a few drops of
    Tabasco or Worcester
    sauce

SERVES 1
5–6 MINS TO MAKE

Eggs can get boring – this keeps them interesting and tasty.

⊃·⊛·○·⊃·⊛·○

Heat the oil in a frying pan and, once hot, add the beaten eggs to the pan, along with the parsley, spring onion and tomatoes (if you want them cooked). Stir everything around in the pan to scramble. Add salt and pepper to taste, then put all except half a handful of the spinach leaves into the pan. Allow to wilt and mix into the scrambled eggs. Once cooked to your desired consistency, serve the scramble on top of the remaining (uncooked) spinach leaves, with a dash of Worcester or Tabasco sauce, if you like.

FRUITY QUINOA WITH HOME-ROASTED ALMONDS

¾ cup cooked quinoa
1 cup fresh berries (any)
½ banana
1 kiwi fruit
2 tbsp roasted almonds*
juice of ½ a lemon
½ tsp natural honey

SERVES 1
7–15 MINS TO MAKE

Quinoa is a good alternative to cereal and is gluten free. As a bonus, it tastes great savoury or sweet.

Put the quinoa in a bowl and toss with the berries. Peel and slice the banana and kiwi fruit into the bowl. Then sprinkle the roasted almonds on top. Squeeze over the fresh lemon juice and drizzle with the honey.

TIP

Home-roasted almonds can be made beforehand and kept in an air-tight container. They will last a couple of weeks. Roasting enhances the natural sweetness of nuts.

1–2 bags plain almonds

Preheat the oven to 100°C/gas ¼. Lay a sheet of greaseproof or baking paper on a baking tray. Spread the almonds evenly over the paper. Place in the preheated oven for 7–15 minutes (depending how roasted you like the almonds to be). Remove from the oven and leave to cool.

 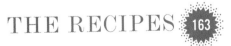

7 SUPERFOODS CEREAL

2 tbsp ground flaxseed mix
    (any brand will do, but we
    prefer Linwoods, which
    has sesame and sunflower
    seeds and goji berries)
1 tbsp desiccated coconut
1 tsp ground cinnamon
1 tbsp chia seeds
½ cup frozen or fresh
    blueberries
½ cup frozen or fresh
    raspberries
¼–½ cup just-boiled water
1–2 tsp manuka or
    natural honey

Cereal toppings:
1 banana, chopped
oat or almond milk
    (as needed)

SERVES 1
3–5 MINS TO MAKE

This is gluten free with no wheat grains, but has plenty of good fibres and good fats from the flaxseed and chia seeds.

Place all the dry ingredients and the berries in a small to medium-sized saucepan. Pour over enough boiling water to combine the ingredients but not so much that the mixture is swimming or totally covered in water. Slowly simmer the ingredients, allow the 'porridge' to heat through and the berries to defrost (if frozen). Add the honey and continue to keep moist by adding a little water, as required, as it cooks and heats through. You'll notice the chia seeds become gelatinous – this holds the mixture together like sticky porridge.

Serve once you feel it's made to your liking (after 3–5 minutes usually). Top with chopped-up banana and oat milk or almond milk, as desired.

SALMON & SCRAMBLED EGGS

2 eggs
1 tsp organic butter
Pink Himalayan salt
    and freshly ground
    black pepper
2 slices of smoked salmon
    or 1 small fillet of fresh
    steamed/baked salmon

SERVES 1
3–4 MINS TO MAKE

This is my absolute favourite Saturday morning breakfast. It has good fats from the salmon and protein from eggs, which sets you up for the day.

Whisk the eggs and set aside. Then melt the butter in a frying pan. Once the pan is hot enough and the butter is sizzling, pour the beaten eggs into the pan and stir to scramble as they cook. Season with salt and pepper and serve with a side of smoked or cooked salmon.

BE BODY
BEAUTIFUL

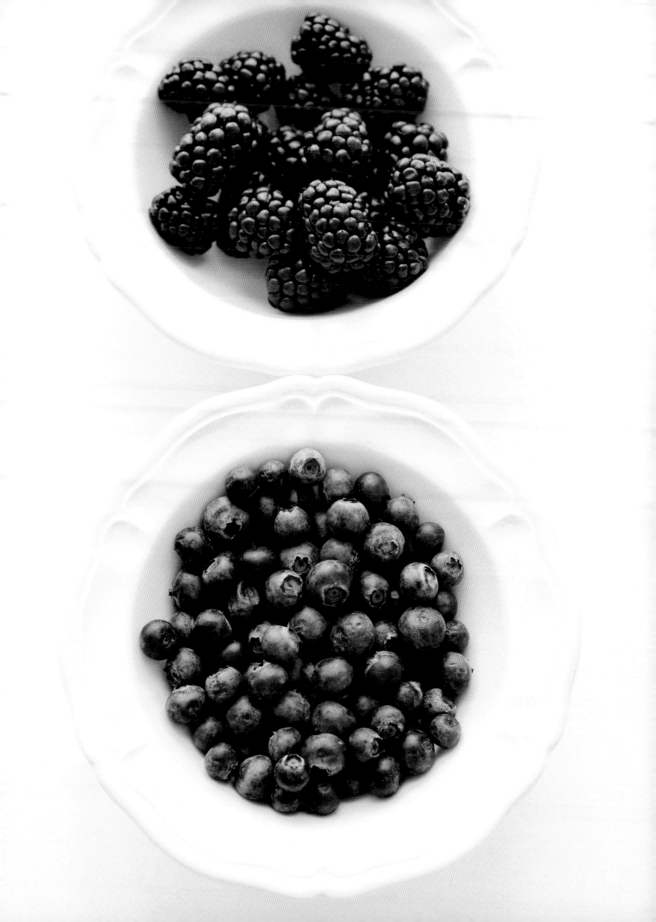

GRATED CARROT, CASHEW & RAISIN SALAD

2–3 large carrots, peeled
¼ cup raisins
½ cup raw cashew halves
2 tbsp olive oil
2 tbsp apple cider
1 tbsp apple cider vinegar
½ tsp curry powder
½ tsp freshly grated ginger
a dash of ground cinnamon
salt and freshly ground black
   pepper, to taste

SERVES 4–5 AS A SIDE DISH
6–7 MINS TO MAKE, PLUS
1 HOUR CHILLING TIME

This is so fresh and delicious. I feel like I'm on holiday whenever I eat it!

Slice the carrots into long ribbons with a vegetable peeler straight into a large bowl. Add the raisins and the cashews. In a separate small bowl, combine the olive oil, cider, cider vinegar, curry powder, ginger and cinnamon by whisking vigorously.

Add a little salt and pepper to taste, whisk again and then pour the dressing over the salad. Gently toss everything to combine, then cover and place in the refrigerator for 1 hour prior to serving.

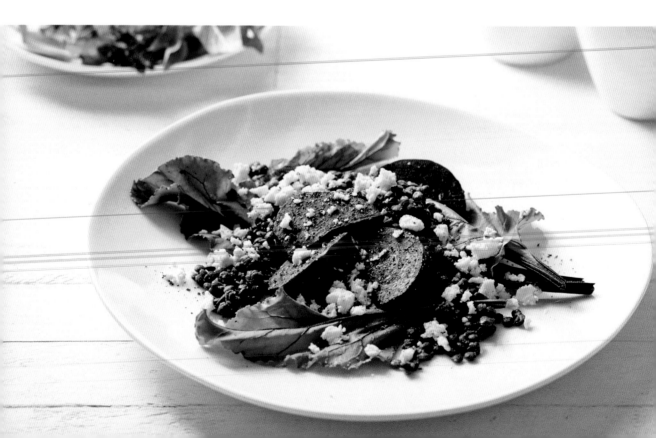

FENNEL & WALNUT SALAD

a 1cm piece of fennel, chopped
1 small carrot, peeled and
finely chopped
¼ of a purple or green
cabbage, finely shredded
1 spring onion, chopped
1 celery stick, chopped
½ cup walnut pieces

For the dressing:
a splash of extra virgin
olive oil
a couple of fresh mint
leaves, ripped
cayenne pepper, to taste
1 garlic clove, peeled and
minced or crushed
optional: 1tbsp flaxseeds

SERVES 1–2
5–6 MINS TO MAKE

Nuts in moderation are very good for you, and walnuts in particular are great for brain function.

Mix all the salad ingredients together in a bowl. Make the dressing by whisking those ingredients together in a separate small bowl, then tip over the salad as required, and toss to coat.

BEETROOT & EGG SALAD

3 medium cooked beetroots,
cut into quarters
2 hard-boiled eggs, peeled
and cut into quarters
1 handful rocket or baby
lettuce leaves
1 tsp savoury seed mix
1 tbsp olive oil
1 tbsp balsamic vinegar

SERVES 1
10 MINS TO MAKE

This is a really tasty lunch option. Beetroot is brilliant for boosting iron and tastes scrummy.

Combine all the salad ingredients together in a bowl and then dress with the oil and vinegar.

 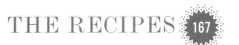

STICKY EGG & AVOCADO SALAD

**2 medium-boiled eggs,
    peeled and diced**
**1 medium avocado, peeled
    and diced**
**a handful of fresh spinach
    leaves**
a drizzle of olive oil
a drizzle of balsamic vinegar
freshly ground black pepper

SERVES 1
7–10 MINS TO MAKE

Eggs and avocado are a good match. They
are high in protein and healthy fats.

Sliced tuna makes a delicious and healthy
addition to any salad.

Mix the eggs, avocado and spinach together in a
bowl, drizzle with the oil and vinegar, then grind on
some pepper. Toss the salad in its dressing and enjoy.

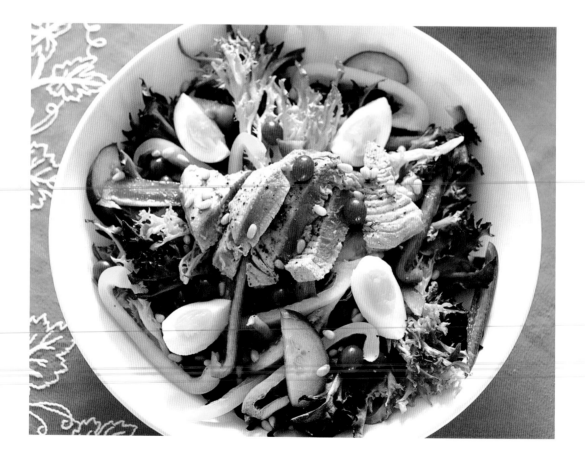

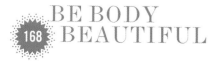
BE BODY
BEAUTIFUL

SUPERFOOD SALAD/
GRAIN-FREE SUPERFOOD SALAD

a handful of baby
　spinach leaves
a handful of kale, very
　finely chopped
a handful of fresh coriander
　or mint, very finely chopped
　(other herbs which work
　well are parsley and basil)
1 large tomato or 8 small
　cherry tomatoes, sliced
　or diced
¼ of a cucumber, diced
½ an avocado, peeled and
　sliced or diced
2 tbsp natural seed mix (most
　supermarkets do one)
optional: 4 pieces of jarred
　artichoke hearts
optional: ½ cup cooked
　quinoa, brown rice or
　buckwheat (N.B. This can
　be taken out of the recipe
　to make it a grain-free
　superfood salad.)
optional: 1 tbsp feta
　cheese chunks
　(for a veggie version)
optional: ½–1 cooked chicken
　breast or 1–2 cooked
　chicken thighs (for a
　non-veggie version)

SERVES 1
5 MINS TO MAKE

This is so good for you. Quinoa and buckwheat make sure that this salad is wonderfully filling, meaning you won't need to snack later. It's also really tasty.

Combine all the ingredients in a bowl and serve.

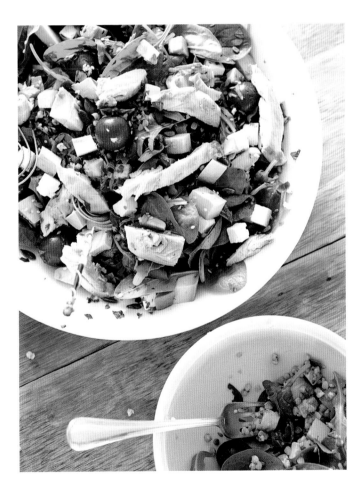

FENNEL MIXED SALAD

½ a small bulb of fennel, chopped
1 small carrot, peeled and
    finely chopped
a handful of purple cabbage
    leaves, chopped
1 spring onion, chopped
1 celery stick, chopped

Dressing:
a splash of extra virgin olive oil
2 fresh mint leaves, finely
    chopped
cayenne pepper, to taste
1 garlic clove, peeled and minced
    or very finely chopped
optional: 1 tbsp flaxseeds

SERVES 1
7 MINS TO MAKE

Fennel has quite a strong taste but it is
detoxifying and SO good for you.

Put all the salad ingredients in a bowl and mix
together. Make the dressing in a separate small
bowl, pour over the salad and toss to coat.

SPINACH, APPLE & WALNUT SALAD

2 Golden Delicious apples,
    cored and cut into large dice
4 tbsp lemon juice
8 cups baby spinach leaves
    (approx. 1 large 300g bag)
3 tbsp extra-virgin olive oil
1 tbsp apple cider vinegar
2 tbsp honey
salt and freshly ground pepper,
    to taste
⅓ cup crumbled goat's cheese
½ cup chopped toasted walnuts

SERVES 4
4–5 MINS TO MAKE

This is a great taste combo – the apple and
walnut are delicious together.

Toss the apple cubes with 2 tablespoons of the lemon
juice in a small bowl. Place the spinach in a large bowl
and remove any long stems or bruised leaves. Whisk
together the remaining lemon juice with the olive oil,
vinegar, honey and some salt and pepper. Toss
together the spinach with the apples and dressing,
then divide between four bowls. Top with the cheese
and walnuts.

BE BODY
BEAUTIFUL

PICK 'N' MIX LUNCH SALAD

1 carrot, peeled and grated
    or chopped
1 avocado, peeled and sliced
5–6 cherry tomatoes, cut in half
a handful of spinach leaves
a small handful of fresh parsley
a small handful of macadamia
    nuts
juice of ½ a lemon
1 tbsp apple cider vinegar

*You can pick from the below
to add some variety:*
for extra greens, add cooked
    broccoli, asparagus or green
    beans, steamed parsnips/
    turnips or boiled/grated
    beetroot
for added protein and really
    healthy fat, try adding line-
    caught tuna or oily fish such
    as mackerel
a hard-boiled egg or some grilled
    chicken is also a great way of
    getting protein into your meal
fruits: such as berries, melon or
    grapefruit
nuts: such as almonds or walnuts
cheese: full-fat feta, mozzarella,
    blue cheese or Brie
meats/fish: cooked chicken,
    beef, turkey, (cured) ham,
    cooked sardines, salmon,
    cod, halibut or snapper
add any vegetable you can
    imagine
Experiment, experiment,
    experiment! Variety is
    the spice of life!

SERVES 2
6–7 MINS TO MAKE

I like days where I can mix it up and this salad allows you to chose exactly what you fancy. Anything goes.

The key here is to be flexible – it's called Pick 'n' Mix for a reason. Whatever's in your fridge and is fresh, go for it.

⋆ ● ◦ ● ⋆ ●

Wash, chop, splash and enjoy.

TIP
This recipe will serve 2, however, by adding whatever you have in the fridge, you could increase the portion size to 4 or more, depending on how many ingredients you use.

 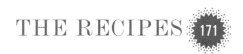

SUSHI SALAD

1 salmon fillet
salt and pepper, to taste
1 tsp coconut oil
½ an avocado, peeled and diced
½ a carrot, peeled and grated
½ a cucumber, grated
1cm ginger, peeled and grated
2 Japanese nori sheets,
   broken into pieces
a handful of beansprouts
1 tbsp tamari sauce (non-
   fermented soy sauce)

SERVES 1
10–12 MINS TO MAKE

I adore sushi, and seaweed is great for minerals
– another great beauty food.

Sprinkle the salmon with salt and pepper and cook
in the coconut oil in a frying pan on a low heat for
4 minutes on each side. Then leave to cool. Mix
together the rest of the ingredients in a bowl and
add the cooled salmon on top.

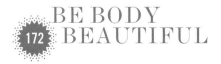

RAINBOW SLAW

3 cups sliced, shredded or
grated cabbage (preferably
half thinly sliced and
half grated)
1 cup grated carrots
(about 1 large carrot)
¾ cup grated cucumber
(skin on)
½ cup thinly sliced sweet onion
¼ cup grated sweet onion
1¼ cups finely chopped flat-leaf
parsley (stems too!)
½ cup shelled organic
hemp seeds
optional: ½ cup chopped
walnuts or pecans and/or
raisins or dried cranberries
1–2 ripe avocados, stoned,
peeled and cut into chunks,
to garnish

*For the tahini dressing (makes
about 1 cup, so refrigerate what
you don't use for later):*
¼ cup tahini
2 garlic cloves, peeled and
crushed
½ cup fresh lemon juice
(about 2 lemons' worth)
¼ cup nutritional yeast,
or a bit more to taste
2–4 tbsp extra-virgin
olive oil, to taste
1 tsp kosher salt and freshly
ground black pepper,
or to taste
3 tbsp water, or as needed
to get a good consistency

SERVES 2-3
5 MINS TO MAKE

It's vibrant, coulourful and high in antioxidant
and powerful cleansing properties from the
cabbage.

The slaw is pretty simple to make. Just grate or
chop all the salad ingredients, put everything in
a giant bowl and toss the veggies together. Put all
the dressing ingredients into a food processor and
process until smooth. Drizzle half the dressing over
the salad and toss again. Garnish generously with
the chunks of ripe avocado and serve.

 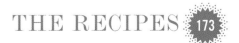

BUTTERNUT SQUASH
& GINGER SOUP

2 rounded tsp organic butter
1 red onion, peeled and
roughly chopped
1 whole garlic bulb, each
individual clove peeled
and cut in half lengthways
5cm ginger root, peeled
and thinly sliced
freshly boiled water
1 litre vegetable or chicken
stock (homemade, or
shop-bought is fine)
1 medium swede, peeled
and diced
2 medium butternut squashes,
peeled and diced
½ tsp pink Himalayan salt
Greek yogurt, to serve
a handful of baby spinach
leaves, chopped

SERVES 4 (SO SHARE WITH
THE FAMILY OR REFRIGERATE/
FREEZE LEFTOVERS)
30 MINS TO MAKE

A great winter warmer.

In a stock pot or large saucepan, gently melt the
butter over a low heat. Add the onion, garlic and
ginger to the pot and shallow fry. If they start to stick,
pour in a little bit of freshly boiled water to allow the
vegetables to continue to cook. Once they have
softened, add the stock and bring to the boil gently.
Next, add the diced swede and squash to the soup
mix, season with the salt and pour in more boiled
water – enough to cover the contents by about 2–3cm.
Leave to simmer for 20 minutes, until the vegetables
are soft, checking the water level every so often. Turn
off the heat and, using a blender (a hand-held one is
ideal), purée to create a smooth soup. Serve in bowls
with a dollop of Greek yogurt and a sprinkling of
chopped baby spinach leaves.

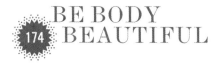

CHICKEN, STRAWBERRY & KIWI SALAD

½–1 cooked chicken breast
(baked or, ideally, steamed)
75g fresh organic strawberries,
hulled and diced
2 handfuls of baby spinach
leaves, shredded
1 kiwi fruit, peeled and sliced
pink Himalayan salt and black
pepper, to season

For the dressing:
2 tsp balsamic vinegar
2 tsp extra virgin organic
olive oil
1 tsp sesame oil (or just
use olive oil)
1 tsp natural honey

SERVES 1–2
5 MINS TO MAKE

This is a great summery salad, especially
with a BBQ.

Toss all the salad ingredients together in a bowl.
Combine all the dressing ingredients in a clean jam
jar, screw on the lid and shake well. Pour the dressing
over salad just before serving, and season with salt
and pepper.

TAHINI DRESSING

1/4 cup tahini
2 garlic cloves
1/2 cup fresh lemon juice
(about 2 lemons)
1/4 cup nutritional yeast
or a bit more, to taste
2–4 tbsp extra virgin olive oil,
to taste
1 tsp kosher salt and freshly
ground black pepper,
or to taste
3 tbsp water, or as needed

MAKES 1 CUP
5 MINS TO MAKE

A creamy way to jazz up salad.

In a food processor add all ingredients and process
until smooth.

 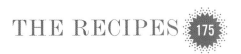

CARROT, CASHEW & CHILLI SOUP

8–10 medium carrots,
   peeled and finely diced
2 garlic cloves, peeled
   and crushed
1 tbsp olive oil
a pinch of sea salt
freshly ground black pepper
50g cashew nuts or 2 tbsp
   natural peanut butter
750ml–1 litre vegetable stock
a pinch of chilli powder
a handful of fresh mint
   leaves, chopped
juice of 1 lime

SERVES 4 (SO SHARE WITH
YOUR FAMILY OR REFRIGERATE/
FREEZE LEFTOVERS)
45 MINS TO MAKE

Gorgeous. The creamy thickness combined with the metabolism-boosting chilli makes for an irresistable winter warmer.

Preheat the oven to 220°C/gas 8 and place a roasting tin in the oven to heat up. Put the carrots, garlic and olive oil in the hot roasting tin, then season with salt and pepper. Roast in the preheated oven until the carrots are tender enough to mash – about 20 minutes.

If using cashews, spread them out evenly on a sheet of greaseproof or baking paper on a baking tray. Place in the preheated oven until they are golden (around 5 minutes). Remove from the oven and leave to cool. Mix in a food processor or using a pestle and mortar until the mixture is like peanut butter (or just use natural peanut butter, if preferred).

Heat your stock. Once the carrots are cooked, mash together with the nut butter and a few splashes of the stock until you have a thick, smooth and creamy mash. Add a hint of chilli powder, to taste. Mix in the fresh mint to counter the heat from the chilli. Trickle and mix in enough stock to get the soup as thick or thin as you like. Season again to taste and finish with a refreshing squeeze of lime juice.

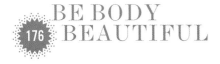

ASPARAGUS & ARTICHOKE SOUP

1 jar of artichoke hearts
1 tbsp organic butter
1 medium shallot or 1 small
    green onion, peeled
    and chopped
1 bunch of asparagus, ends
    discarded then chopped
1 x 400g tin of water
    chestnuts, drained
    and sliced
1 tsp vegetable stock powder
1 tbsp fresh tarragon leaves
    or 1½ tsp dried tarragon
3 cups filtered water
¼ cup raw macadamia or
    cashew nut butter
pink Himalayan salt and
    freshly ground black
    pepper
10 sprigs of fresh watercress

SERVES 4–6 (SO SHARE WITH
YOUR FAMILY OR REFRIGERATE/
FREEZE LEFTOVERS TO
USE LATER)
30 MINS TO MAKEW

This is a favourite of mine. I love the flavours, and the green veg is a bonus.

Chop the artichokes coarsely and set aside. Put the butter, shallot or onion and asparagus in a saucepan over a low heat. Mix and sauté gently for 4–5 minutes.

Add the artichokes, water chestnuts, stock powder and tarragon leaves and then heat through. Add about 2 cups of water to the vegetables. Meanwhile stir the remaining cup of water into the nut butter until smooth, and then carefully stir into soup. Stir the soup frequently while warming over a medium-low heat until the mixture is heated through. Do not boil.

Taste for seasoning. Serve the soup chunky or blend until smooth, if preferred. Pour into bowls then top with the watercress.

 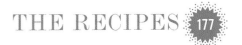

HEARTY VEGETABLE SOUP

4 courgettes
3 tomatoes
2 celery sticks
a small handful of green beans
3 garlic cloves, peeled
1 small onion, peeled
4 cups water
sea salt
chopped fresh parsley and
    coriander to garnish

SERVES 4–6 (SO SHARE WITH
YOUR FAMILY OR REFRIGERATE/
FREEZE LEFTOVERS TO USE LATER)
30 MINS TO MAKE

A classic vegetable soup that is easy, quick
and tasty.

Chop up the vegetables and put into a saucepan
along with the water. Bring to the boil and simmer
until all the vegetables are cooked. (Try not to
overcook them, but leave the veggies a little bit
crunchy if you can.)

Season with a little salt to taste. Either drain the broth
and serve the vegetables separately, or blend to make
a thick soup. Serve in bowls, garnished with the herbs.

THAI FISH SOUP

1 tbsp coconut oil
2.5cm ginger, peeled and grated
1 lemongrass stem, finely cut
1 red chilli, finely cut
5 cups vegetable or fish stock
1 red pepper, seeded and sliced
3–4 pak choi
juice of 2 limes
1 tbsp fish sauce
1 tbsp Tamari (healthy
    alternative to soy sauce)
1½ cups coconut milk
2 fish fillets (e.g. cod, halibut,
    snapper), cut into large chunks

SERVES 4 (SO SHARE WITH YOUR
FAMILY OR REFRIGERATE/FREEZE
LEFTOVERS TO USE LATER)
10–15 MINS TO MAKE

This warming soup reminds me of being in
Thailand. The flavours make my mouth water.

Put the coconut oil, ginger, lemongrass and chilli
into a large pan on a low heat for a few minutes.
Add the rest of the ingredients (except the fish).
Cook until the vegetables are soft, then add the fish
chunks. Leave to simmer and serve the soup when
the fish is cooked through.

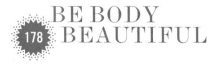

BE BODY
BEAUTIFUL

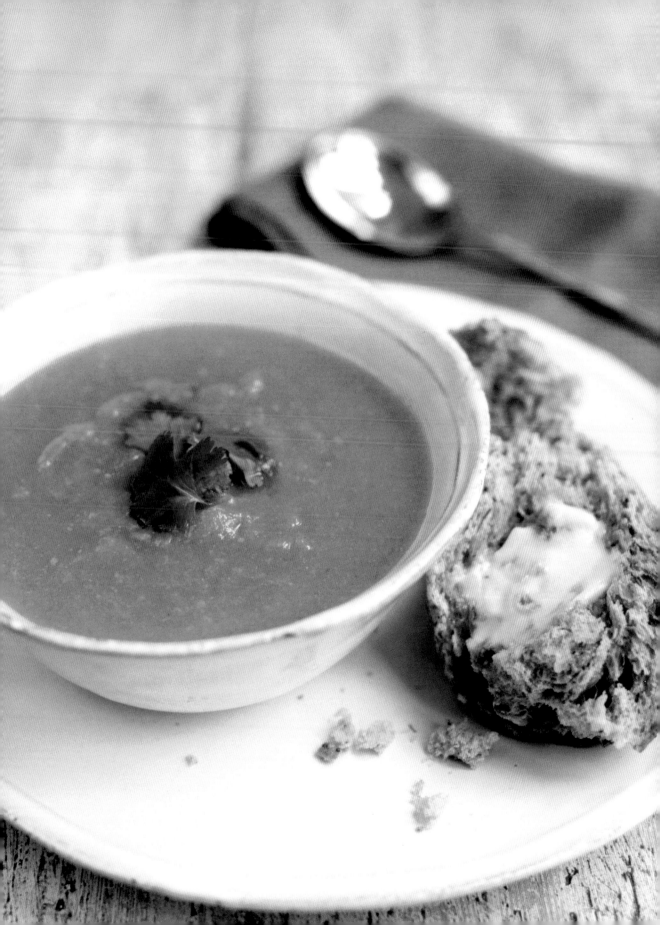

CARROT & CORIANDER SOUP

2 tbsp coconut oil, ghee
or butter
2 onions, peeled and chopped
6 garlic cloves, peeled
and chopped
3 carrots, peeled and
chopped
1 medium sweet potato,
peeled and cuts into cubes
8 cups vegetable stock
1 tsp ground cumin and/
or turmeric
salt and cayenne pepper,
to taste
½ cup chopped fresh parsley
chopped fresh coriander,
to taste

SERVES 2
30 MINS TO MAKE

Coriander is very cleansing, as well as delicious.

Put the oil, ghee or butter in a medium-large
saucepan over a low heat. Add the onion and garlic
to the pan and sweat until they soften.

Then add the carrots and sweet potatoes, stir and
leave to sauté for a few minutes. Pour in the vegetable
stock and turn up the heat.

Add the cumin and/or turmeric. Bring the soup to
a boil and let it simmer until the vegetables are soft.
Season with salt and cayenne pepper, then add the
parsley. Blend, then pour the soup into bowls and
serve with some chopped coriander sprinkled on top.

GREEN SOUP

1 tbsp coconut oil
1 courgette, chopped
2 garlic cloves, peeled
and chopped
½ a green cabbage, chopped
1½ cups water or
vegetable stock
a handful of spinach leaves
a large handful of fresh
parsley
juice of 1 lemon

SERVES 1–2
15 MINS TO MAKE

Vegetables are key for a healthy, happy diet,
so load up on this.

Put the oil in a saucepan over a low heat, then add
the courgette, garlic and cabbage. Cook until just
softened, then add the water or stock. Bring to a
simmer but don't overcook the vegetables. Add the
spinach, parsley and lemon juice and blend when
the mixture has cooled a little.

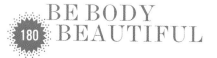

COURGETTE & MINT SOUP

4 tbsp olive oil
a generous knob of butter
1 small onion, peeled
   and chopped
2 small courgettes,
   thinly sliced
a pinch of salt
300g frozen peas
500ml vegetable stock
a handful of mint, torn
a handful of watercress,
   chopped
50g spreadable goat's cheese
8 small pieces of toasted
   sourdough bread

SERVES 3–4 (SO SHARE WITH
THE FAMILY OR REFRIGERATE/
FREEZE LEFTOVERS)
[TIME] 10–12 MINS TO MAKE

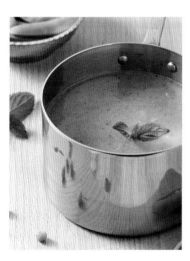

An irresistable superfood soup.

Put half the oil and all the butter into a saucepan on
a medium heat. Add the onion and sauté until soft,
but without colour, then put the courgettes into the
pan, season with salt and cook for about five minutes.
Stir in the peas, pour in the stock (topping it up with
water to cover the veggies if necessary), bring to
the boil, and simmer for a few minutes. Check the
seasoning, then blend the mixture to make a smooth
soup, thinning it with a little water if needed.

If you prefer the soup cold, pour it into a container
with ice cubes to chill quickly, then cover and
refrigerate. Chill your serving bowls before pouring
in the soup, and garnish with a sprinkling of the mint
and watercress and drizzling over the remaining olive
oil. Spread the goat's cheese on to the sourdough
toast to make croutons and serve these on the side.

 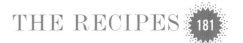

FEEL-GOOD VEGGIE SOUP

4 courgettes
3 tomatoes
2 celery sticks
a small handful of green
  beans, trimmed
3 garlic cloves, peeled
1 small red or white
  onion, peeled
4 cups water
sea salt
chopped fresh parsley and
  coriander, to garnish

SERVES 2–4
15 MINS TO MAKE

This is a really delicious soup, and a tasty way to get your five a day in one bowl!

⊙·⊙·⊙·⊙·⊙·⊙

Chop all the vegetables and put in a saucepan with the water. Bring to the boil and simmer until everything is cooked (but try not to overcook the vegetables, leaving a little bit of crunch and goodness). Season with salt. Either drain the broth and serve the vegetables separately, or blend together to make a thick soup. Serve in bowls, garnished with the herbs.

MACA DIP

2 tbsp plain Greek yogurt
2 tsp maca powder
1 tbsp ground flaxseeds
1 apple or 1 banana, sliced

SERVES 1
2–3 MINS TO MAKE

Maca balances hormones and tastes naturally sweet.

⊙·⊙·⊙·⊙·⊙·⊙

In a bowl, combine the yoghurt, maca powder and ground flaxseeds. Mix together and serve with the sliced fruit.

BE BODY
BEAUTIFUL

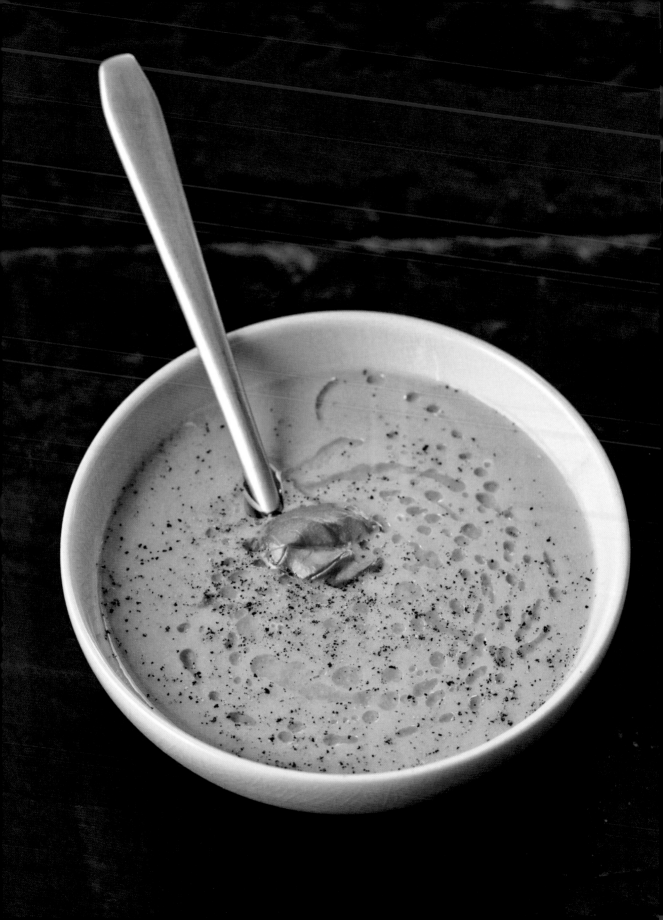

SALMON NORI ROLLS

2 tsp horseradish
2 Japanese nori sheets
  (seaweed paper/sushi paper)
2 slices of smoked salmon or
  1 small fillet of steamed/
  baked then chilled fresh
  salmon, halved (leftovers
  can be used)
1 small carrot, peeled and grated
¼ of a cucumber, thinly sliced
dark soy sauce (make sure it's
  MSG free!), to serve

SERVES 1
5–6 MINS TO MAKE

Superfoods all rolled into one – seaweed, avocado and salmon all provide healthy fats.

Spread 1 teaspoon of horseradish over each nori sheet. On one end layer a piece of salmon, some grated carrot and a few slices of cucumber. Then tightly roll the nori sheet up and lightly wet the inside of the last bit so that the nori sticks and the roll stays complete. Repeat to make a second roll with the remaining ingredients. Serve with the soy sauce as a dipping sauce.

VEGETABLE & CASHEW NORI ROLLS

2 Japanese nori sheets
  (seaweed paper/sushi paper)
4 tsp jarred cashew butter
  or crushed cashew nuts
optional: 2 tsp horseradish, if
  using crushed cashews (they
  need something to stick to)
1 small carrot, peeled and grated
¼ of a cucumber, thinly sliced
¼ of a avocado, peeled and
  thinly sliced
a squeeze of lemon juice
optional: ¼ of a red chilli,
  deseeded and finely chopped
dark soy sauce (make sure
  it's MSG free!), to serve

SERVES 1
5–6 MINS TO MAKE

A tasty vegetarian option, and the cashew nuts are a great source of healthy fats.

Spread 2 teaspoons of cashew butter (or 1 teaspoon of horseradish if using instead) over each nori sheet. Layer the vegetables at one end and sprinkle over the chopped cashews (if using). Squeeze on some lemon juice and sprinkle over a little chopped chilli, if you like. Then tightly roll up each nori sheet around the filling, and lightly wet the inside of the last bit of nori so that it sticks and the rolls stay together. Serve with soy sauce as a dipping sauce.

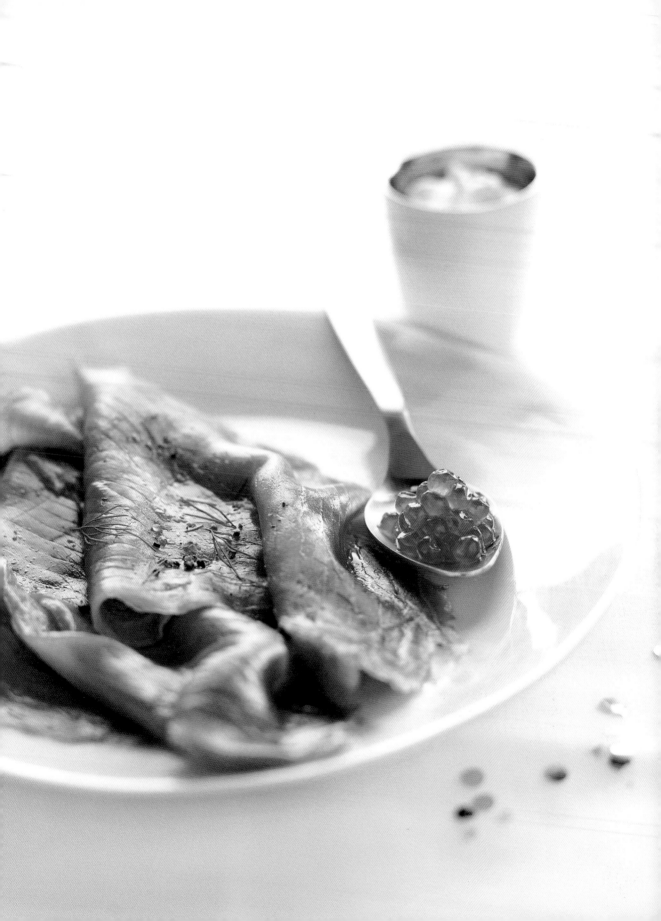

SEAWEED ROLLS

2–4 Japanese nori sheets
    (seaweed paper/sushi
    paper), 2 per person
1 carrot, peeled and grated
¼ of a lettuce, shredded
½ an avocado, peeled and
    cut into long, thin slices
100g raw or cooked salmon
    or cooked beef slices
optional extras: cucumber
    slices, wasabi/mustard

SERVES 1–2
4–5 MINS TO MAKE

Seaweed is packed full of minerals that nourish
your body.

Place the ingredients in neat lines along the nori
sheets. Roll up each nori tightly to ensure the filling
doesn't fall out.

PEA & PARSLEY CREPE

5–6 handfuls of baby
    spinach leaves
¼ cup frozen peas
pink Himalayan salt and
    freshly ground black
    pepper, to season
3 large eggs
¼ cup rice or almond milk
coconut oil, for sautéing
¼ cup finely chopped
    flat-leaf or curly parsley
avocado salsa or guacamole,
    to serve (pages 205
    and 208)

SERVES 1–2
5–7 MINS TO MAKE

This is something a little bit different and
a good way to get the kids to eat their peas!

Wilt the spinach in a large non-stick saucepan for
a few minutes and drain. Add the peas to the same
pan as the spinach and gently cook. Remove from
the heat and season with salt and pepper.

Whisk the eggs and milk together. Heat a little
coconut oil in a medium frying pan and pour in the
egg mixture. As the eggs just begin to set, sprinkle
them with the chopped parsley. Tip the spinach and
peas in the middle. When the bottoms of the eggs
are lightly browned, gently roll the egg over into
a roll. Then serve with salsa or guacamole.

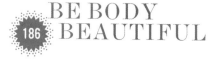

PALEO PLATE

2 hard-boiled eggs, peeled
a handful of nuts
    (your choice)
guacamole salsa twist
    (page 208)

SERVES 1
3 MINS TO MAKE

This meal will fire up your metabolism and keep hunger at bay. Perfect for keeping carbs low and protein high.

· · · · · ·

Arrange the ingredients on a plate and dig in!

SPICED VEGETABLE QUINOA

3 tbsp coconut oil
1 large onion, peeled
    and finely chopped
2 garlic cloves, peeled
    and crushed
1 tbsp tomato purée
½ tsp ground turmeric
½ tsp cayenne pepper
1 tsp ground coriander
1 tsp ground cumin
1½ cups cauliflower florets
1 red pepper, seeded and diced
2 courgettes, sliced
1 x 400g tin of chickpeas,
    drained and rinsed
4 beefsteak tomatoes,
    skinned and sliced
pink Himalayan salt and
    freshly ground black pepper
2 cups quinoa
a handful of chopped
    fresh coriander

SERVES 6–8 (SO SHARE WITH
YOUR FAMILY OR REFRIGERATE/
FREEZE LEFTOVERS)
25–30 MINS TO MAKE

I love quinoa because it can be savoury or sweet. It fills you up, too, like rice, but is much better for you!

· · · · · ·

Heat 2 tablespoons of the oil in a large pan, add the onion and garlic, and cook until translucent. Stir in the tomato purée and spices, and continue to cook, stirring well, for 2 minutes. Add the cauliflower and red pepper with enough water to come halfway up the vegetables. Bring to the boil, lower the heat, cover and simmer for 10 minutes. Add the courgettes, chickpeas and tomatoes to the pan and cook for a further 10 minutes. Season then keep the spicy vegetables warm, ready to serve shortly.

To cook the quinoa, bring a saucepan full of water to the boil. Add the quinoa and stir. Bring back to the boil and simmer for 10–12 minutes, or until the quinoa is soft. Serve on plates topped with the vegetable curry mixture and sprinkle on the fresh coriander.

 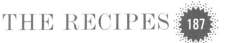

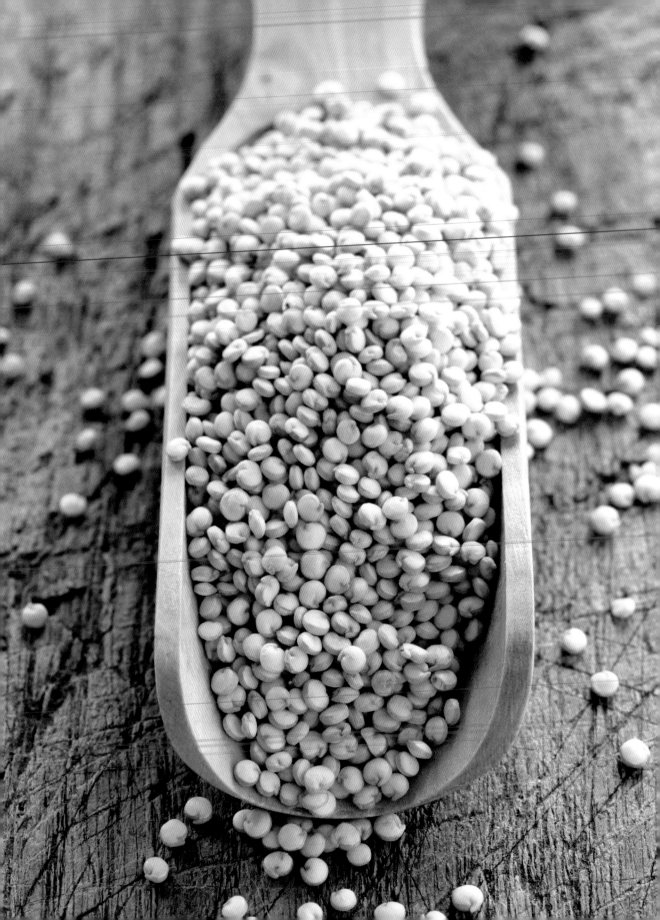

CANNELLINI BEAN & QUINOA PATTIES

a knob of coconut oil or
   organic butter, for frying
   (N.B. If frying with butter,
   always have a dash of water
   ready to add to it, to stop
   it burning.)
½ a red onion, peeled
   and finely chopped
1 garlic clove, peeled
   and crushed
½ tsp fennel seeds, crushed
2 tsp ground cumin
1 x 400g tin of cannellini
   beans, drained and rinsed
1 cup cooked quinoa
1 egg, beaten
a handful of chopped parsley
a handful of spinach leaves,
   finely chopped
pink Himalayan salt
   and freshly ground
   black pepper

MAKES 10–12 PATTIES
(SO SHARE WITH THE FAMILY
OR REFRIGERATE/FREEZE
LEFTOVERS)
12–15 MINS TO MAKE

A healthy and delicious alternative to meat patties.

Heat the coconut oil or butter in a large frying pan over a medium heat. Sauté the onions for a few minutes, until soft, and then add the garlic and spices. Cook for a minute, or until aromatic, then tip in the cannellini beans. Toss them well in the oil and spices until coated and then turn off the heat.

Mash the beans roughly with a potato masher and then add the quinoa, egg, parsley and spinach. Season well with salt and pepper and give everything a good mix – use (clean) hands if necessary. Form the mixture into 10–12 small rounds and press down so that the patties are about 2.5cm thick. I find it easiest to use a lever ice-cream scoop to scoop out the mixture for even-sized patties and then I press lightly with the palm of my hand to flatten them slightly. Fry the patties for a few minutes each side in a lightly coconut-oiled frying pan over a medium heat, until golden and heated through. Be careful as you turn the patties, as they can be a little fragile.

Serve with sides of hummus, tzatziki, homemade relish or salsa.

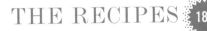

STEAMED MEDITERRANEAN COD

1 x 400g tin of chopped
   tomatoes
a pinch of natural salt
½ a red or yellow pepper,
   seeded and sliced
1 tsp capers
1 clove garlic, peeled
   and crushed
a handful of chopped
   Mediterranean herbs (such
   as basil and/or oregano)
1–2 cod fillets

SERVES 1–2
10 MINS TO MAKE

Cod is such a versatile fish. It is high in protein
and soaks up flavours well.

In a saucepan, heat the chopped tomatoes, and
add the salt, sliced pepper, capers, crushed garlic
and herbs. Heat the mixture through until it reaches
simmering point, then cook for 5 minutes until
the flavours combine.

Meanwhile, steam the cod fillet(s) for 5 minutes
or until just cooked. Serve the cod with steamed
vegetables and pour over the tomato sauce.

TURKEY & CHICKPEA CURRY

1 x 400g tin of chickpeas,
   drained, rinsed
500g turkey escalopes/
   breasts, cut into thin strips
1 red onion, peeled and sliced
1 x 400g tin of chopped
   tomatoes
a pinch of saffron
1 cinnamon stick
½–1 tsp chilli powder
a pinch of pink Himalayan salt
½ tsp ground cumin
½ cup buckwheat

SERVES 3–4 (SO SHARE WITH
YOUR FAMILY OR REFRIGERATE/
FREEZE LEFTOVERS)
45 MINS TO MAKE

The spices are all cleansing and nourishing, and
this dish is great for winter. It's a guilt-free Friday
night curry . . .

Preheat the oven to 180°C/gas 4. Put all the
ingredients (except the buckwheat) into a casserole
dish and mix well, ensuring the turkey and chickpeas
are fully covered in liquid. Cook in the preheated
oven for 30–35 minutes. Meanwhile, cook the
buckwheat in boiling water for 10–15 minutes until
soft. Drain and rinse in boiling water. Serve the curry
on top of the buckwheat with plenty of steamed
mixed green veg on the side.

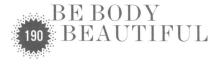

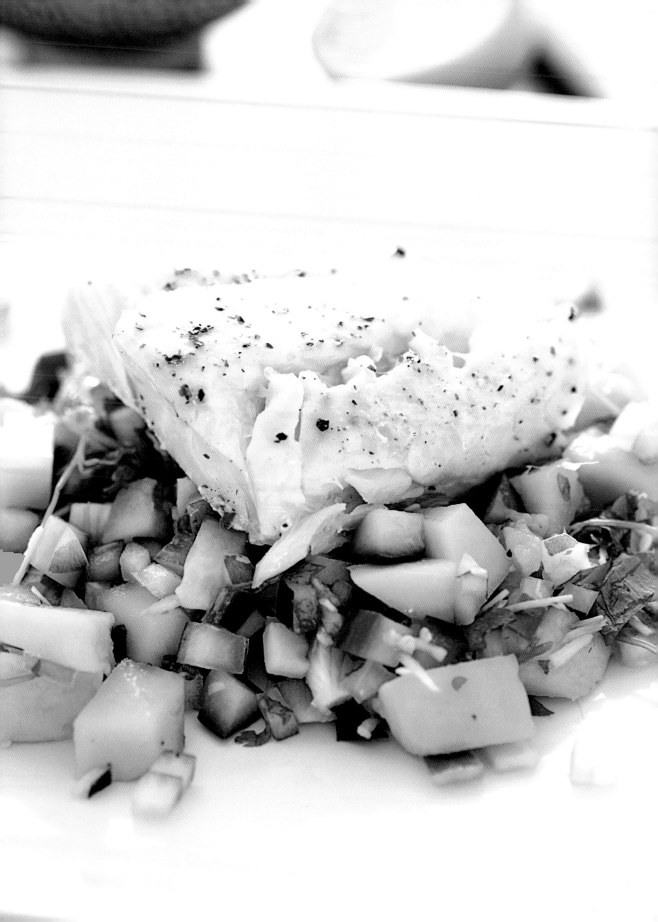

VEGAN CHICKPEA & PARSNIP CURRY

1 cup dried chickpeas,
  soaked in water over
  night, or 1 x 400g tin
  of chickpeas, drained
  and rinsed
7 garlic cloves, peeled
  and finely chopped
1 small onion, peeled and
  finely chopped
5cm fresh root ginger,
  peeled and chopped
2 small green chillies,
  chopped
450ml plus 5 tablespoons
  water
1 tbsp coconut oil
1 tsp cumin seeds
2 tsp ground coriander
1 tsp ground turmeric
1 tsp chilli powder or
  mild paprika
½ cup ground cashew nuts
250g tomatoes, peeled
  and chopped
900g parsnips, peeled
  and cut into chunks
Celtic sea salt and black
  pepper, to taste
1 tsp ground cumin
juice of 1 lime
chopped fresh coriander,
  to serve

SERVES 3–4 (SO SHARE WITH
THE FAMILY OR REFRIGERATE/
FREEZE LEFTOVERS)
30–40 MINS TO MAKE, PLUS
1¼–1¾ HOURS IF USING DRIED
CHICKPEAS

A super-high protein dish. Good on a workout day.

If using dried chickpeas, put the soaked chickpeas in a pan, cover with cold water and bring to the boil. Boil vigorously for 10 minutes, then reduce the heat and boil steadily. Cook for 1–1½ hours, or until the chickpeas are tender. Drain and set aside.

Keep 2 teaspoons of the chopped garlic to one side, then blend the remainder in a food processor with the onion, ginger and half the chopped chillies. Add 5 tablespoons of water to the mixture and blend again until you have a smooth paste.

Heat the oil in a large frying pan and cook the cumin seeds for 30 seconds. Stir in the ground coriander, turmeric, chilli powder or paprika and the ground cashew nuts. Add the paste to the pan and cook, stirring frequently, until the water begins to evaporate. Add the tomatoes and fry for 2–3 minutes. Next add the cooked or tinned chickpeas and parsnip chunks to the mixture with the 450ml of water, a little salt and plenty of black pepper. Bring to the boil, stir, then simmer, uncovered, for 15–20 minutes, until the parsnips are completely tender. If the curry seems too watery, turn up the heat and boil fiercely until the sauce is thick. Add the ground cumin with a little more salt and the lime juice, to taste. Stir in the reserved garlic and green chilli, and cook for a further 1–2 minutes.

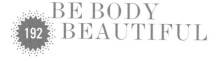

BEEF & TOMATO COCONUT CURRY

1 tbsp olive oil
500g lean casserole
  steak, diced
1 red onion, peeled
  and chopped
1 red chilli, seeded and sliced
2 large garlic cloves, peeled
  and finely chopped
5cm ginger, peeled and
  finely sliced
1 lemongrass stem, outer
  leaves removed and
  chopped
1 x 400ml tin of coconut milk
1 x 400g tin of chopped
  tomatoes
300ml beef stock
1 cinnamon stick
1 star anise
a handful of chopped
  fresh coriander
salt and pepper
1 aubergine, chopped

SERVES 3–4
2 HOURS TO MAKE

Too delicious for words. I LOVE it.

Preheat the oven to 160°C/gas 3. In a casserole dish, heat the oil over the hob and brown the steak (in batches if necessary). Set aside. Soften the onion in the casserole dish and stir in the chilli, garlic, ginger and lemongrass and cook for 1 minute. Return the steak to the pan and stir in the coconut milk, tomatoes and stock.

Stir in the other spices and the coriander, then season. Bring to the boil, cover and then put in the preheated oven for about 1 hour 45 minutes. Stir in the aubergine halfway through cooking.

 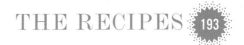

CAULIFLOWER & CHICKPEA CURRY

2 cups chickpeas, soaked in
    filtered water overnight
2 tbsp coconut oil
1 large onion, peeled
    and finely chopped
5 garlic cloves, peeled,
    crushed and finely
    chopped
½ a large cauliflower,
    trimmed and cut into
    bite-sized pieces
2 tbsp ground turmeric
2 tbsp cayenne pepper
salt and pepper, to taste
2 cups coconut milk

SERVES 4 (SO SHARE WITH
YOUR FAMILY OR REFRIGERATE/
FREEZE LEFTOVERS TO
USE LATER)
25 MINS TO MAKE

A tasty, nourishing curry that is brimming
with flavour.

⊃ · ⊕ · ⊂ · ⊃ · ⊕ · ⊂

Drain and rinse the soaked chickpeas. Fast boil for
ten minutes and slow cook for up to an hour. Put the
coconut oil and onion into a large saucepan over
a medium heat.

Once the onions are golden, add the garlic. Cook
for ½–1 minute, then add the cauliflower and
chickpeas. Add the spices to the pan, stir to coat,
season with salt and pepper and cook for 3–4
minutes, stirring regularly.

Pour in the coconut milk, bring to a simmer and
leave for 10–15 minutes, or until the cauliflower is
cooked. Serve on a bed of steamed green vegetables.

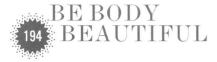

PACIFIC ISLAND FISH CURRY

a pinch of sea salt

1½ tbsp tamarind paste,
dissolved in a cup of water
(if you can't find tamarind
paste an alternative is to
squeeze the juice of a lime
into the water)

500g meaty white fish (such
as cod), cut into chunks

1 x 400ml tin of coconut milk

juice of 1 lemon

For the curry paste:

1 tbsp coconut oil

1 onion, peeled and finely
chopped

3 garlic cloves, peeled,
crushed and finely chopped

2 tbsp garam masala or
mixed spice

1 tbsp ground turmeric

1 tsp cayenne pepper

1 tsp ground cumin

zest of 1 unwaxed lemon

a big bunch of coriander,
ripped or finely chopped
(save a bit for sprinkling
on top of the curry)

SERVES 4 (SO SHARE WITH YOUR
FAMILY OR REFRIGERATE/FREEZE
LEFTOVERS TO USE LATER)
10 MINS TO MAKE

A delicious way to eat fish – even if you don't
usually love fish this will take your fancy.

First make the curry paste. Put the coconut oil
and the onion into a large frying pan and cook until
golden. Add the rest of the curry paste ingredients
and stir over a medium heat for around 2 minutes.
Blitz the paste in a blender, if you like, but it's
not essential!

Stir the salt and tamarind liquid into the curry paste
in the pan. Add the fish and mix with the paste. Pour
in the coconut milk and bring everything to a simmer
for 2–4 minutes, or until the fish is completely cooked
through. Serve sprinkled with the reserved coriander,
a squeeze of lemon juice and extra salt to taste. This
curry goes well with quinoa and green beans.

TIP

Add more water to the curry to get it to the
consistency that you want, but don't add too
much that you dilute the flavour.

 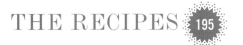

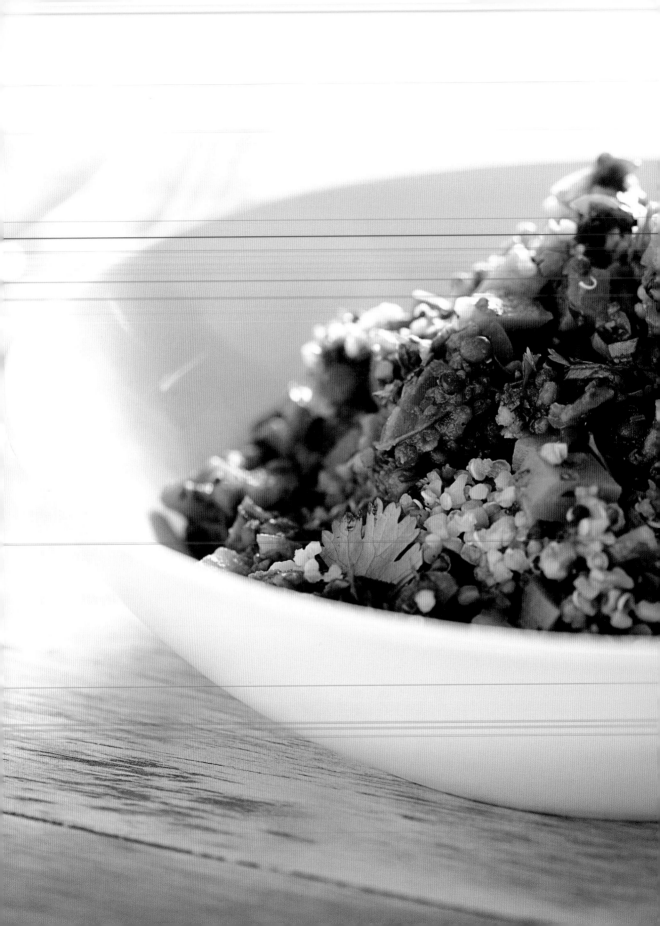

LENTIL BOLOGNAISE

2 cups cooked green lentils
  (prepared as per packet
  instructions)
2 garlic cloves, peeled,
  crushed and diced
1 small onion, peeled
  and finely diced
2 tomatoes, finely diced
½ a red pepper, seeded
  and chopped
1 carrot, peeled and chopped
1 celery stick, chopped
a handful of fresh parsley,
  roughly chopped
a handful of fresh coriander,
  roughly chopped
cayenne pepper, to taste
salt and pepper, to taste

SERVES 4 (SO SHARE WITH
YOUR FAMILY OR REFRIGERATE/
FREEZE LEFTOVERS)
30 MINS TO MAKE

Perfect if you want the comfort of bolognaise without the meat!

Blend half of the lentils until smooth and put both the whole and blended lentils aside. Then put the garlic and onion in a non-stick pan, and cook until golden then add the tomatoes.

Meanwhile, boil the rest of the vegetables separately, but make sure to leave them still slightly crunchy. Put all the ingredients together in one big pot and add the herbs and seasoning. Serve with buckwheat or brown rice.

 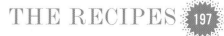

THREE BEAN VEGGIE CHILLI

1 tbsp coconut oil or
   organic butter
1 large carrot, peeled and diced
1 large celery stick, diced
1 medium onion, peeled and
   finely chopped
1 garlic clove, peeled and
   finely chopped
optional: 1 red chilli, finely
   chopped, or ½–1 tsp
   chilli powder
1 tbsp tomato purée
1 tsp ground cumin
1 tsp ground coriander
1 bay leaf
1 cinnamon stick or a piece
   of cassia bark
1 tsp smoked paprika
1 x 400g tin of chopped tomatoes
1 red, green or yellow pepper,
   seeded and chopped
1 tsp soy sauce
1 x 400g tin of kidney beans,
   drained and rinsed (or 100g
   dried beans, soaked overnight
   and cooked as per the packet
   instructions)
1 x 400g tin of adzuki beans,
   drained and rinsed (or 100g
   dried beans, soaked overnight
   and cooked as per the packet
   instructions)
1 x 400g tin of black-eye beans,
   drained and rinsed (or 100g
   dried beans, soaked overnight
   and cooked as per the
   packet instructions)
a handful of fresh coriander
   leaves, chopped

This is very high in protein and it's a good healthy option when you are hungry.

Put the oil or butter in a large, wide pan on a medium heat. Add the carrot, celery, onion, garlic and fresh chilli (if using) and sweat until the onions are translucent – about 10 minutes. Add the tomato purée and stir for 30 seconds, then add the cumin, ground coriander, bay leaf, cinnamon stick or cassia bark, smoked paprika and dried chilli (if using). Fry the spices for a minute, before adding the chopped tomatoes, chopped pepper and soy sauce. (Adding the pepper at this stage leaves it with a bit of crunch. If you like it softer, then add along with the carrot and onion.) Bring everything to a simmer, cover and leave on a low heat for 10–20 minutes, stirring occasionally, until the veg are cooked through.

Tip in the three sorts of beans, stir the chilli, bring it back to simmering point and cover. Cook over a low heat for a further 10–15 minutes, until the beans are hot. Keep an eye on the mixture, adding a couple of tablespoons of water if it is a bit dry. Stir in the chopped coriander leaves just before serving.

SERVES 4 (SO SHARE WITH
THE FAMILY OR REFRIGERATE/
FREEZE LEFTOVERS
[TIME] 40–50 MINS TO MAKE

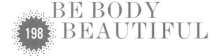

VEGGIE CHILLI

1 medium–large onion,
   peeled and chopped
1 tbsp coconut oil
several garlic cloves, peeled
   and crushed or finely
   chopped (quantity as
   per your taste)
1 finely chopped fresh chilli,
   or 1 tsp chilli paste
   or powder
1 x 400g tin of butter
   beans, rinsed
1 x 400g tin of kidney
   beans, rinsed
1 x 400g tin of chickpeas,
   rinsed
6 medium tomatoes, diced
1 cup passata (or just blend
   some fresh tomatoes
   yourself)
optional: a good glug
   of decent red wine

SERVES 4 (SO SHARE WITH
THE FAMILY OR REFRIGERATE/
FREEZE LEFTOVERS)
30 MINS TO MAKE

A healthy alternative to chilli con carne.

Fry the onion in the coconut oil in a large pan for a
few minutes, until slightly golden. Add the garlic and
chilli and let those cook for about 30 seconds. Then
tip in the beans and chickpeas, mix and cook for
a couple of minutes.

Add the tomatoes and passata. Add enough water
to give the desired consistency, bring to the boil then
simmer gently for around 15-20 minutes. This is
where the red wine goes in, if using, so you can keep
it separate from any kids' portions.

After adding the wine, cook the chilli for a further 5
minutes, then serve on a bed of buckwheat or quinoa.

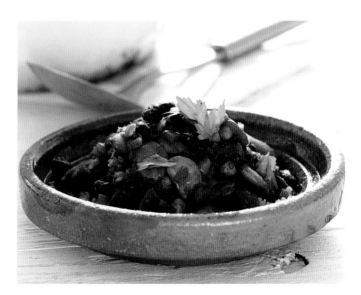

 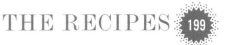

TARRAGON TURKEY BURGERS

aubergine, cut into 4 x
   1cm-thick round slices
optional: organic butter
olive oil
Celtic sea salt
3 grinds of black pepper
450g minced turkey
55g grated courgette
30g chopped red onion
1 tbsp fresh or dried
   tarragon leaves
2 tsp Dijon mustard
½ tsp vegetable seasoning
   (e.g. Oxo cube) or salt
2 large eggs, beaten
butternut squash, peeled
   and cut into 4 x 1cm-thick
   round slices
organic cranberry sauce

SERVES 4 (SO SHARE WITH
YOUR FAMILY OR REFRIGERATE/
FREEZE LEFTOVERS)
20 MINS TO MAKE

Tarragon is a delicious herb, and these burgers are a nice change from a traditional beef pattie.

Preheat the oven to 180°C/gas 4. Blanch the aubergine slices in a saucepan of boiling water for up to 1 minute. Remove from the water and lay on a baking tray either greased with butter or lined with baking paper. Brush both sides of each aubergine slice generously with olive oil and season with salt and pepper. Bake in the preheated oven for around 10–15 minutes, until soft and brown, turning them over half way through the cooking time.

Meanwhile, in a mixing bowl, combine the turkey mince with the courgette, onion, tarragon, mustard, seasoning (or salt) and eggs. Mix thoroughly. Shape into 4 patties and grill in the oven (once aubergine has been removed) until cooked. Steam the squash slices until soft all the way through – but do not allow them to go soggy, as they need to keep their form.

Make the stacks from the bottom up: first a squash slice, then an aubergine one, followed by the burger and a little cranberry sauce. Serve with a generous side salad, including lots of leaves.

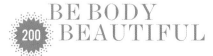

BEEF BURGERS

500g lean steak mince
½ a red onion, peeled
   and finely chopped
1 egg, beaten
1 tsp dried oregano
1 garlic clove, peeled
   and crushed
1 tbsp Worcester sauce
1 tsp soy sauce
1 tbsp tomato paste
optional: butter or coconut
   oil, for frying

For the sweet potato fries:
2–3 medium-sized sweet
   potatoes
2 tbsp chilli oil (chilli-
   infused olive oil)
½ tsp pink Himalayan salt
several grinds of black
   pepper, to season
a pinch of bouillon
   or stock powder

SERVES 4 (SO SHARE WITH
THE FAMILY OR REFRIGERATE/
FREEZE LEFTOVERS)
45–50 MINS TO MAKE

You don't have to buy frozen burgers. You can easily make these for the kids and they are really tasty and healthy.

Start by making the sweet potato fries. Preheat the oven to 180°C/gas 4 and wash and peel the sweet potatoes. Cut them into fry-shaped slices, then put the sweet potato slices in a large self-seal plastic bag and add the remaining sweet potato fries ingredients to the bag. Seal the bag, or tie the top into a knot to seal, and shake until all of the sweet potatoes are evenly coated. Pour out the slices on to a baking tray lined with greaseproof or baking paper. Bake in the preheated oven for 40–45 minutes, or until browned on the outside, turning them halfway through. Meanwhile, combine all the burger ingredients in a bowl with your hands until evenly mixed. Roll approximately half a tablespoon of the mince mixture into a ball in the palm of your hands (you shouldn't need flour to prevent it sticking as the tomato paste will do this) and then squash into a patty of your desired thickness. Grill the patties for 15 minutes (turning as needed) under a medium–high grill. Serve with salad and the sweet potato fries, which go well with plain unsweetened yogurt as a dipping sauce and tomato salsa. (These are healthy versions of those typical chip accompaniments, mayonnaise and ketchup!)

 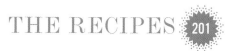

GRILLED MACKEREL FILLETS WITH APPLE CHUTNEY

4 x 250g mackerel fillets,
   filleted and boned
olive oil
½ tsp cayenne pepper
½ tsp thyme leaves
baby spinach leaves , to serve
2 limes, cut into wedges

For the chutney:
1 small onion, peeled and
   finely chopped
a pinch of ground cumin
a pinch of cumin seeds
a pinch of ground ginger
a pinch of ground turmeric
a pinch of chilli powder
1 garlic clove, peeled and
   finely chopped
coconut oil, for frying
250g cooking apples, peeled
   and roughly chopped
2 tbsp cider vinegar
2 tbsp natural honey
1 tsp hazelnut (or any nut) oil

SERVES 4 (SO SHARE WITH
YOUR FAMILY OR REFRIGERATE/
FREEZE LEFTOVERS)
25 MINS TO MAKE

Mackerel is an oily fish that is a fantastic source of omega-3 and high in protein. It's great after an evening workout.

To make the chutney, sweat the onion with all the spices, garlic and a little coconut oil in a stainless steel pan for 2 minutes over a medium heat. Add the apples to the pan, together with the rest of the chutney ingredients, and simmer over a low heat for 20 minutess.

Meanwhile, lightly brush the mackerel fillets with olive oil and sprinkle with the cayenne pepper and thyme. Place on a grilling tray. Grill the mackerel under a hot grill for 8 minutes until golden brown. Cook the spinach in a large saucepan until slightly wilted. Serve the fish on a bed of the spinach, with a spoonful of the chutney on top. As always, additional salad vegetables on the side are recommended.

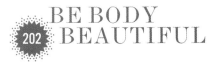

HOMEMADE BEEF BOLOGNAISE

1 red onion, peeled and
   finely chopped
3 garlic cloves, peeled
   and finely chopped
1 organic beef stock cube
3 large bay leaves
125ml red wine
300–500g organic
   minced steak
2 tbsp tomato purée
1 x 400g tin of chopped
   tomatoes
½ tsp pink Himalayan salt
freshly ground black pepper
a pinch of dried oregano

SERVES 3–4 (SO SHARE WITH
YOUR FAMILY OR REFRIGERATE/
FREEZE LEFTOVERS)
25–30 MINS TO MAKE

A perfect weekend treat and a family favourite!

Start cooking the onion, garlic and stock cube in
a saucepan in a small amount of boiled water (just
enough to cover the base of the pan). Add the bay
leaves and allow the water to simmer gently. Once
you can smell the bay leaves, add the red wine and
bring the mixture to simmer again. Add the minced
meat and start immediately breaking it down until
the mince and the wine become a sauce together.

As the liquid reduces and the mince starts to cook,
mix in the tomato purée and the chopped tomatoes.
Once the meat is cooked through, season with salt
and pepper, and the dried oregano.

 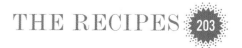

BASIC DHAL

3 tsp organic butter or ghee
1 onion, peeled and chopped
2 green chillies, seeded
  and chopped
1 tsp chopped fresh ginger
55g dried yellow or red
  lentils, rinsed
900ml filtered water
3 tbsp roasted garlic purée
  (paste) or 4 garlic cloves,
  peeled and crushed
1 tsp ground cumin
1 tsp ground coriander
Sea salt and freshly ground
  black pepper
200g tomatoes, peeled
  and diced
a little lemon juice
a few fresh coriander leaves

SERVES 2-3 (SO SHARE WITH
YOUR FAMILY OR REFRIGERATE/
FREEZE LEFTOVERS)
30 MINS TO MAKE

This is a classic Indian dish, so tasty and full of fibre.

Melt the butter or ghee in a pan, add the onion, chillies and ginger and cook for 10 minutes until golden. Stir in the lentils and water, bring to the boil, then reduce the heat and partly cover. Simmer, stirring occasionally, for 50–60 minutes, until it has a very thick, soup-like consistency.

Stir in the roasted garlic purée or crushed garlic, cumin and ground coriander. Season with salt and pepper and cook for a further 10–15 minutes uncovered, stirring frequently. Then stir in the tomatoes, adjust the seasoning to your taste and add lemon juice as you like it. Serve, sprinkled with fresh coriander leaves.

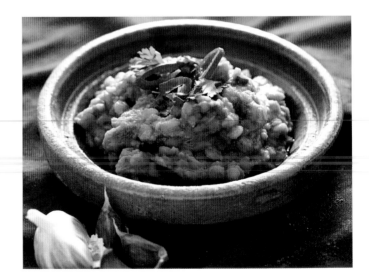

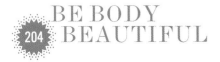

BLACK BEAN PATTIES

1 onion, peeled and
   finely chopped
1 red pepper, seeded
   and finely chopped
1 x 400g tin of black beans,
   drained and rinsed
2 garlic cloves, peeled
   and minced
1 cup cooked quinoa
a small handful of parsley,
   finely ripped
a sprinkle of ground cumin
coconut oil, for frying

For the avocado salsa dip:
1 ripe avocado
2 radishes, finely chopped
juice of 1 lemon

SERVES 4 (SO SHARE WITH
YOUR FAMILY OR REFRIGERATE/
FREEZE LEFTOVERS)
10 MINS TO MAKE

An alternative to beef patties. The dark beans look the part and taste delicious. They're high in protein and full of fibre too.

Brown the onion in a little olive oil in a pan and then add the red pepper, black beans and garlic. Cook for 2 minutes then add the cooked quinoa, parsley and cumin. Tip the mixture from the pan into a blender and blend together until well combined. Remove from the blender and, once slightly cooled, form into 4 palm-sized patties (if you make them all the same thickness that will ensure even cooking). Shallow fry the patties in coconut oil in a frying pan for 4 minutes on each side, or until cooked through.

To make the avocado salsa dip, loosely mash the avocado flesh in a small bowl, add the radishes and squeeze on lemon juice. Mix well together. Serve the black bean patties with the dip.

TIP

Ensure the patties are well compacted before cooking, otherwise they will break apart.

 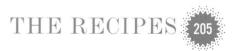

SPICED CHICKEN OR CHICKPEA CASSEROLE

1 x 400g tin of chopped
   tomatoes
1 onion, peeled and
   finely chopped
1tsp ground cumin
1tsp ground turmeric
½–1 tsp chilli powder
1 star anise
1 cinnamon stick
¼ tsp pink Himalayan salt
4 chicken thighs (with or
   without skin and bones)
   or 1 x 400g tin of organic
   chickpeas

*Requires slow cooker
   or casserole dish.*

SERVES 3-4
1 HOUR 45 MINS TO MAKE

A classic dish, great for the slow cooker. Put it on before you leave the house and in the evening it's all ready for you.

⊹⊹⊹⊹⊹⊹⊹

If you don't have a slow cooker, preheat the oven to 175°C/gas 4. In a casserole dish or slow cooker, mix together the tomatoes, onion, spices and salt. Add the chicken thighs or chickpeas and push them into the tomato mixture, spooning it over the chicken so each piece is covered. Cover with a lid and slow cook for 8 hours on low or bake in the preheated oven for 1½ hours, or until the chicken is cooked through and tender. You'll know the chicken is cooked when it separates easily from the bone, or it simply flakes in half when pressed. Let the casserole stand for 10–15 minutes before serving with mixed steamed vegetables or a clean carb (as instructed on your meal planner).

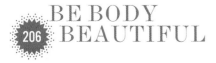

BEAUTY BOWL

½ cup cooked and cooled
     quinoa or buckwheat
½ cup steamed broccoli
     or cauliflower
1 cup finely chopped steamed
     greens (kale, spinach,
     chard, etc)
¼ of a red onion, peeled and
     finely chopped
1–2 small carrots, peeled
     and grated
1–2 celery sticks, chopped
1 garlic clove, peeled and crushed
½ an avocado, peeled and diced

For the dressing:
1 tbsp olive oil
salt
juice of ½ a lemon
a pinch of cayenne pepper

SERVES 2
10 MINS TO MAKE

This is self-explanatory. Eat healthily and you
will glow on the outside.

Mix all the salad ingredients in a big bowl. Whisk
together the dressing ingredients in a separate small
bowl, then drizzle over the salad and toss everything
together before serving.

QUINOA TABBOULEH

2–3 medium tomatoes,
     finely chopped
1–2 small onions, peeled
     and finely chopped
1 celery stick and/or ¼ of
     a cucumber, finely chopped
a big handful of finely chopped
     fresh coriander and parsley
200g cooked quinoa or
     buckwheat
juice of 1 lemon
½ tbsp olive oil
a sprinkle of cayenne pepper

SERVES 2
4–5 MINS TO MAKE

Delicious tabbouleh without the wheat.

Mix all the vegetables, herbs and quinoa or
buckwheat together into a bowl. Squeeze on the
lemon juice, drizzle the olive oil and sprinkle
the cayenne. Toss and serve.

 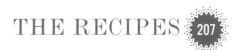

LETTUCE CHICKEN TACOS

500g chicken thighs
2 tbsp coconut oil
salt and pepper, to taste
1 medium onion, peeled
and chopped
1 garlic clove, peeled and
minced
1 red pepper, seeded and diced
1 celery stick, diced
1 iceberg or romaine lettuce
2 spring onions, trimmed
and chopped

*For the guacamole
salsa twist:*
a large handful of baby
spinach leaves
flesh of 2 large ripe avocados,
roughly chopped
juice of 1 lemon
2 tbsp minced fresh parsley,
coriander or dill
salt and freshly ground
pepper, to taste

SERVES 4 (SO SHARE WITH YOUR
FAMILY OR REFRIGERATE/FREEZE
LEFTOVERS TO USE LATER)
40 MINS TO MAKE

Finger-friendly food that is tasty and good for you! Great for a Friday night in with mates.

Preheat the oven to 180°C/gas 4. Cut the chicken thighs into bite-sized strips and put them into a bowl, then add half the coconut oil (1 tablespoon) and plenty of salt and pepper. Mix to coat. Transfer the chicken to a baking tray and put in the preheated oven for 15–20 minutes, or until cooked through and golden on top.

To make the guacamole, put all the guacamole ingredients into a blender and mix to the desired consistency. Put the remaining tablespoon of coconut oil in a pan over a medium heat, add the onion and, when slightly golden, also add the garlic, red pepper and celery. Stir-fry until cooked but you still want to leave some crunch in the veg.

Lay a couple of lettuce leaves on each person's plate and top them with the vegetable mix, chicken, guacamole and, finally, the diced spring onions.

TIP
If you want to do a vegetarian dish then leave out the chicken and add in a lot more vegetables.

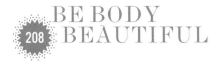
BE BODY
BEAUTIFUL

AUBERGINE CANNELLONI

1 aubergine
sea salt
350g–400g organic
    tomato passata
grated Parmesean cheese

For the filling:
1 cup cooked white beans
    (drained and rinsed
    if from a tin)
a small handful of basil
    leaves
a handful of spinach leaves
2 garlic cloves, peeled
    and crushed
juice of 1 lemon

SERVES 1–2
25–30 MINS TO MAKE

Aubergines are full of vitamins, minerals and fibre and eating them regularly can lower cholesterol.

The aim here is to roll the filling in the aubergine slices, as if they were pasta sheets. Cut the aubergine lengthways into long slices about 2–3mm-thick, lay them in a colander and sprinkle with sea salt. Let the aubergine sit for 10 minutes to get rid of any bitterness. Rinse and dry by blotting with kitchen paper. Then grill the aubergine slices under a medium grill for 5 minutes.

Preheat the oven to 180°C/gas 4. For the filling, mix all the ingredients in a blender. Put a spoonful of the filling on each cooked aubergine slice and roll up. Place the rolls in an ovenproof dish, then cover with the passata and a sprinkling of cheese, and place in the preheated oven until brown on top. Eat the 'cannelloni' with a salad or on its own.

 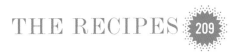

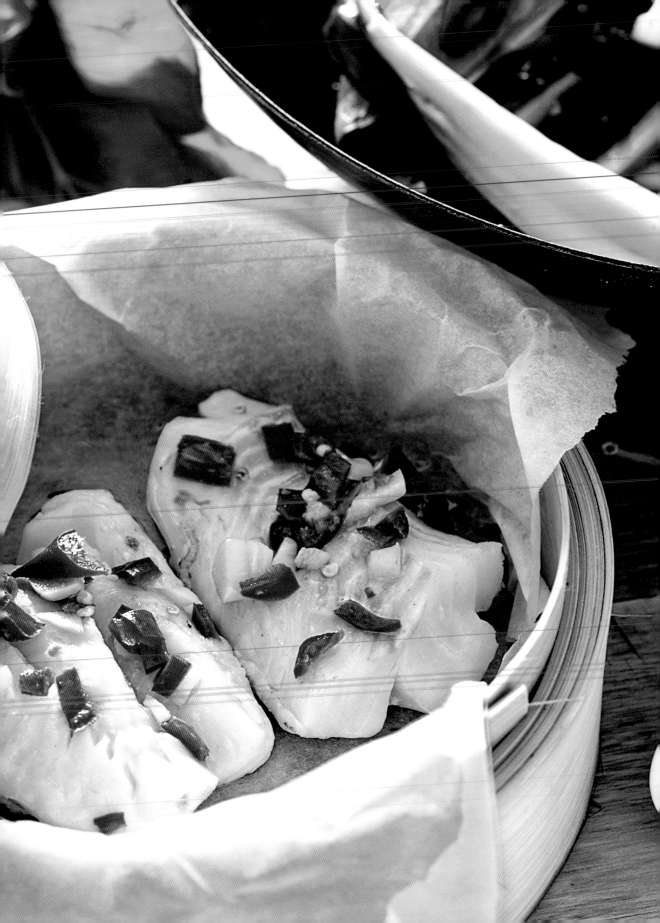

THAI STEAMED FISH WITH ASIAN GREENS

2 trout fillets (or any white fish of your choice)
1cm ginger, peeled and chopped
1 garlic clove, peeled and chopped
1 small red chilli, seeded and finely chopped
juice and zest of 1 lime
3 baby pak choi, quartered lengthways, or 2 normal-sized pak choi, sliced
2 tbsp non-MSG soy sauce
optional: **95g cooked brown rice or quinoa**

SERVES 2
20 MINS TO MAKE

I love the Asian flavours in this dish. Steamed fish is so easy and hassle free.

Lay the fish fillets side by side on a large square of foil and scatter the ginger, garlic, chilli and lime zest over them. Then drizzle the lime juice on top and scatter the pak choi around and on top of the fish.

Pour the soy sauce over the top and loosely seal the foil to make a parcel, making sure you leave space at the top for the steam to circulate as the fish cooks but no liquid should be allowed to leak out of the parcel. Steam the fish parcel for 15 minutes. If you haven't got a steamer, put the parcel on a heatproof plate over a pan of gently simmering water, cover with a lid and steam.

Serve with additional steamed vegetables (such as broccoli, leeks and courgettes) to fill a quarter of your plate, and either brown rice or quinoa. Use the juices from the cooked fish parcel to flavour the rice and other vegetables upon serving.

 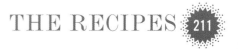

RWL STIR-FRY

a large handful of spinach
    leaves
1 orange or green pepper,
    seeded
1 pak choi
a handful of peeled prawns
    or 200g chicken breast
optional: ¼ cup cooked
    brown rice or 1 cup brown
    rice noodles
1 tbsp coconut oil or ghee

SERVES 2
7–8 MINS TO MAKE

TIP
Add a little soy sauce or
chilli sauce to the stir-fry
to give it some flavour
and juice.

TIP
Add any other vegetables
that you have in the
fridge to your stir-fry,
such as kale and onions,
for example.

This is quick, easy, packed full of nurients
and tastes lovely to boot!

Prepare all the vegetables, and chicken, if using,
by chopping them into bite-sized pieces. If using
noodles, prepare them as per the instructions on
the packet. Put the coconut oil or ghee into a hot
pan (ideally a wok because it is big enough to move
everything around so nothing burns or sticks). Once
the oil is hot enough, add the chicken or prawns to
the pan. Once they have started to change colour, tip
the chopped vegetables in too. Keep the vegetables
moving around and mix with the meat. Cook for
approximately 2–4 minutes, stirring continuously.
If using cooked rice, tip it into the pan to heat through
throughly before serving. Serve the stir-fry either on
top of the noodles on a plate or with the rice mixed
in. Alternatively you can eat it on its own without
noodles or rice.

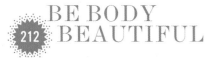

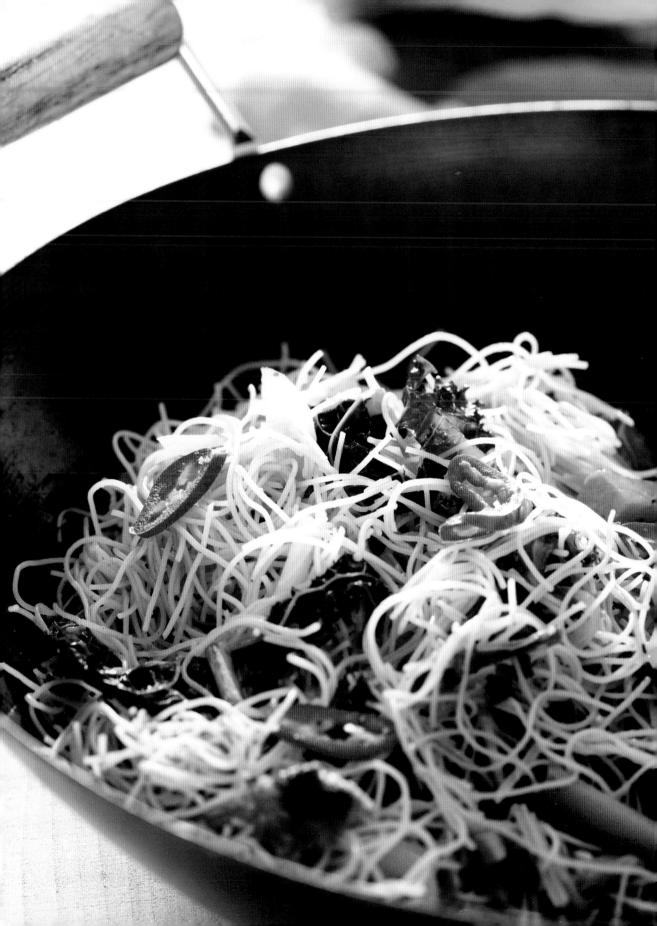

GARLIC ROSEMARY
LAMB CHOPS

1 tsp coconut oil
2 sprigs of rosemary
2 garlic cloves, peeled
  and finely chopped
salt and pepper
4 lamb chops

SERVES 4 (SO SHARE WITH
YOUR FAMILY OR REFRIGERATE/
FREEZE LEFTOVERS TO USE
LATER)
10 MINS TO MAKE

TIP

As a guideline: rare =
2 minutes, medium =
3–5 minutes and well
done = 5–8 minutes (but
depending on the size
and thickness of the meat).
To check, take a sharp
knife and cut into the
middle of the thickest part
of the chop and see if it's
cooked enough for you.

Red meat is a real treat every now and then,
and you can't beat a juicy lamb chop.

Mix the coconut oil, rosemary, garlic, salt and pepper
in a bowl until combined and then massage the
mixture into the chops with your hands.

Place the chops into a hot frying pan or griddle over
a medium–high heat until golden on both sides, then
turn the heat down and cook through as desired. We
suggest a medium chop, so it will be slightly pink in
the centre. Serve with coleslaw and some steamed
broccoli, with roasted vegetables, or on a bed of
quinoa.

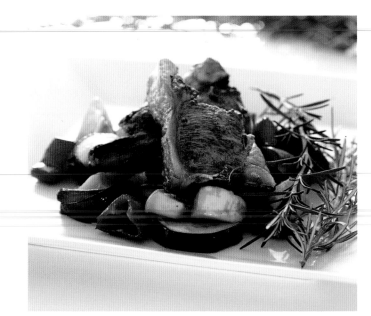

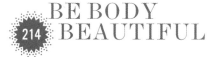

BE BODY
BEAUTIFUL

SALMON WITH OLIVE & GARLIC SAUCE

2 salmon fillets
optional: 1 tsp coconut oil
salt and pepper
2 garlic cloves, peeled
   and finely chopped
juice of 1 lemon
1 tbsp Dijon mustard
2 basil leaves
1 handful of pitted
   olives, halved

SERVES 2
20 MINS TO MAKE

There are so many tasty ways to have salmon, but this is probably my favourite.

Preheat the oven to 180°C/gas 4. Cook the salmon fillets by either steaming them or searing them in a hot pan with the coconut oil until slightly coloured. Then season with salt and pepper and pop them into the preheated oven for 10–15 minutes (depending on the thickness of the fillets).

Meanwhile, cook the garlic by heating it through with the lemon juice in a small pan. Mix together the cooked garlic and lemon juice with the mustard, basil and olives in a bowl. Serve the salmon topped with the garlicky olive mixture, with steamed green vegetables on the side.

TIP
Salmon can be cooked to varying degrees, depending on your preference. In this case, we suggest checking it with a fork to make sure it is a light pink colour all the way through and that the flesh is flaky when you break it apart.

 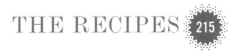

GREEK MEATBALLS

250g minced lamb
250g minced beef
2 tbsp finely chopped
   fresh chives
4 garlic cloves, peeled
   and minced
¼ cup chopped fresh parsley
1 egg, beaten
a handful of fresh mint
   leaves, chopped
1 tsp salt
1½ tsp ground cumin
1 tbsp ground cinnamon
2 tbsp coconut oil
8 sun-dried tomatoes, chopped
8 olives, pitted and chopped

MAKES 12 TO 16 MEATBALLS (SO
SHARE WITH THE FAMILY OR
REFRIGERATE/FREEZE LEFTOVERS)
20 MINS TO MAKE

A real taste of the Mediterranean.

Preheat the oven to 220°C/gas 8. Mix all the ingredients together in a bowl and form into approximately 12 to 16 meatballs with your hands. Place the meatballs on a baking tray lined with greaseproof or baking paper. Put them into the preheated oven and bake for about 15 minutes, depending on size, turning regularly.

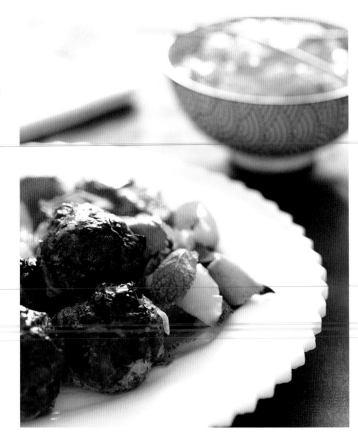

BE BODY
BEAUTIFUL

HEALTHY FISH PIE

2 white fish or smoked
   haddock fillets
2 salmon fillets
1 tsp cumin seeds
1 bag of spinach
1 bag of kale
2–3 handfuls of peeled prawns
1½ cups coconut milk
a small handful of chopped
   fresh coriander
2 tbsp ground turmeric
1 tbsp cayenne pepper, or to
   taste for your preference
   of heat!

For the mash:
1 small–medium butternut
   squash or 4 medium
   sweet potatoes
1 medium cauliflower
a pinch of sea salt and
   black pepper
a small handful of chopped
   fresh parsley
1 tbsp organic butter

SERVES 4 (SO SHARE WITH YOUR
FAMILY OR REFRIGERATE/FREEZE
LEFTOVERS TO USE LATER)
45–50 MINS TO MAKE

Fish is high on the health-food list, but this
feels like a proper tasty and hearty meal.

First, make the mash. Peel and dice the butternut
squash or sweet potatoes and chop the cauliflower.
Boil the vegetables until very soft, then drain the
water from the pan. Season with salt and pepper to
taste, add the parsley and then mash with the butter.
Preheat the oven to 180°C/gas 4. For the filling, steam
all the fish fillets for 7–10 minutes, then gently flake
into chunks and leave to one side. Put the cumin
seeds, spinach and kale, with a splash of water,
in a large saucepan on a low heat, and stir. Once
the leaves are partly wilted, add the rest of the
ingredients (except for the mash) and mix
together thoroughly.

Put the filling mixture into an ovenproof dish, then
top with the mash. Cook in the preheated oven for
10–20 minutes. Serve with optional extra cooked veg
on the side, such as carrots, peas, leeks, etc., or with
a leafy green salad.

 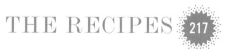

YOGURT WITH PASSION FRUIT & MACADAMIA NUTS

1 cup plain yogurt
2 passion fruits
a small handful of
**   macadamia nuts, crushed**

SERVES 1
2–3 MINS TO MAKE

Just a delicious taste combination. Yogurt is a good replacement for ice cream.

Put the yogurt into a bowl and scoop out the flesh from the passion fruits on top. Swirl through, then sprinkle the crushed macadamias on top.

AVOCADO, CHOCOLATE & STRAWBERRY MOUSSE

2 cups fresh strawberries,
**   plus a few extra to garnish**
flesh of 1 avocado
2 tbsp maple syrup
1 tbsp cocoa powder
2 tbsp water, or more for
**   a texture to your liking**

SERVES 1
4–5 MINS TO MAKE

A guilt-free, dairy-free chocolate mousse.

Blend the two cups of strawberries first. Add the avocado, syrup, cocoa powder and water to the blender, and mix into the strawberries until thick and very smooth. Pour into a bowl. Slice the extra strawberries and use as a garnish when serving the mousse.

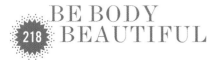

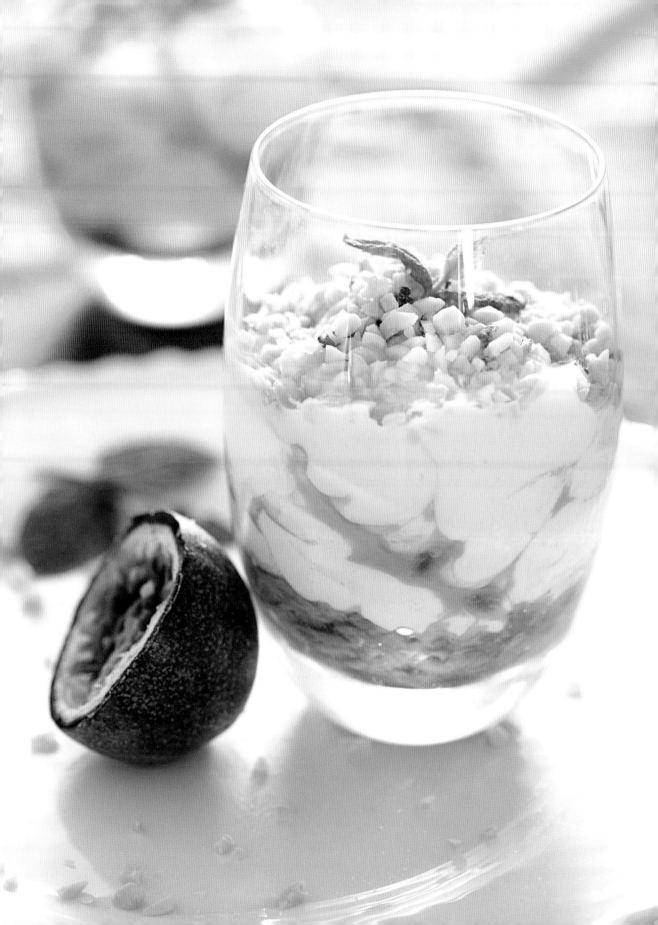

LEMON SORBET

peel of 1 lemon (no pith),
   finely chopped
1 cup filtered water
½ tsp Stevia
½ cup fresh lemon juice
½ cup carbonated
   mineral water
6 strips of lemon peel,
   to garnish

SERVES 6 (SO SHARE WITH
THE FAMILY OR LEAVE IN THE
FREEZER FOR ANOTHER DAY)
15 MINS TO MAKE PLUS 5½
HOURS FREEZING TIME

A refreshing dessert and a great palette cleanser.

In a saucepan, stir together the chopped lemon peel, filtered water and Stevia. Bring to the boil, then reduce the heat to medium and simmer for 5 minutes. Remove the pan from the heat and allow the mixture to cool. Pour the cooled lemon syrup into a jug or bowl and stir in the lemon juice and carbonated mineral water. Pour into an ice-cream maker and freeze according to the manufacturer's instructions. If you do not have an ice-cream maker, you can freeze the mixture in a lidded, deep, freezer-proof plastic container for 1½ hours. Then remove and stir with a whisk. Return the container to the freezer and take it out to stir again once every hour for about 4 hours. The more times you stir, the more air will be incorporated, resulting in a lighter finished sorbet. Remove from the freezer a few minutes before serving to soften slightly. Scoop into bowls and garnish with the strips of lemon peel.

DARK CHOCOLATE SHAKE

flesh of ½ an avocado
flesh of ½ a mango
1 tsp dark organic
   cocoa powder
rice or almond milk
optional: plain organic
   yogurt

SERVES 1
2–3 MINS TO MAKE

A sweet fix without the guilt.

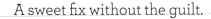

Blend together the avocado and mango flesh with the cocoa powder and the milk in a high-speed blender. If the shake is too thin, mix in a little yogurt (1 tbsp at a time) to get your desired consistency.

BE BODY
BEAUTIFUL

FRESH FRUIT WITH RAW NUT CREAM

1 tsp raw cashew or
    almond butter
1 tbsp plain organic
    Greek yogurt
150–200g fresh fruit (such
    as 1 sliced pear, 1 sliced
    banana, a handful of mixed
    berries or 1 sliced apple)

SERVES 1
3–4 MINS TO MAKE

I love this raw nut and yogurt combo.
The protein makes the fruit more filling.

Mix the nut butter with the yoghurt in a bowl,
then top your fresh fruit salad with this 'cream'.

BERRY MEDLEY WITH COCONUT YOGURT

150g fresh or defrosted
    frozen mixed berries
    (such as raspberries,
    blueberries, blackberries,
    cherries, etc.)
2 tsp desiccated coconut
120ml organic plain or
    Greek yogurt

SERVES 1
2–3 MINS TO MAKE

An antioxidant-rich and guilt-free dessert.

Mix the berries together in a bowl. Stir the coconut
into the yogurt and serve over the berries.

 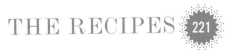

CHIA SEED PUDDING

2 cups almond or rice milk
¼ cup honey, maple syrup
  or agave nectar
2 tsp vanilla extract
½ cup chia seeds

SERVES 1
2–3 MINS TO MAKE, PLUS
4 HOURS CHILLING TIME

Chia is high in protein, fibre and omega-3 and has a perfect consistency for puddings.

ɔ·ø·ɕ·ɔ·ø·ɕ

In a small bowl, whisk together the milk, honey and vanilla. Add the chia seeds and stir to combine. Refrigerate for 4 hours, stirring once halfway through. Serve chilled or allow to warm up to room temperature.

STEWED APPLES WITH YOGURT

1 apple, peeled, cored and
  cut into chunks
a generous pinch of
  ground cinnamon
½ tsp Stevia or honey
1 tsp water
a dollop of plain yogurt,
  to serve

SERVES 1
10 MINS TO MAKE

Apples are such a tasty winter fruit, especially with yogurt instead of cream.

ɔ·ø·ɕ·ɔ·ø·ɕ

Put the apple chunks in a small pan over a low heat and add the cinnamon, Stevia or honey and water. Cover and leave to cook gently, stirring occasionally, until the apple goes mushy. Add a little more water if it seems too dry. Serve warm or cold with a dollop of yogurt on top.

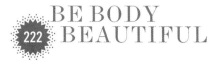

BERRY CRUNCH

1 cup fresh or frozen berries
of your choice (if using
frozen, defrost first)
¼ cup mixed seeds (sesame,
sunflower, pumpkin,
chia and flax)
1 tbsp dried coconut flakes
1 tbsp chopped nuts
(any kind will do)
2 tsp honey or agave nectar

SERVES 1
2–3 MINS TO MAKE

Natural seeds and nuts add some texture
and crunch to the nutritious berries.

Combine all the ingredients in a bowl and
mix thoroughly.

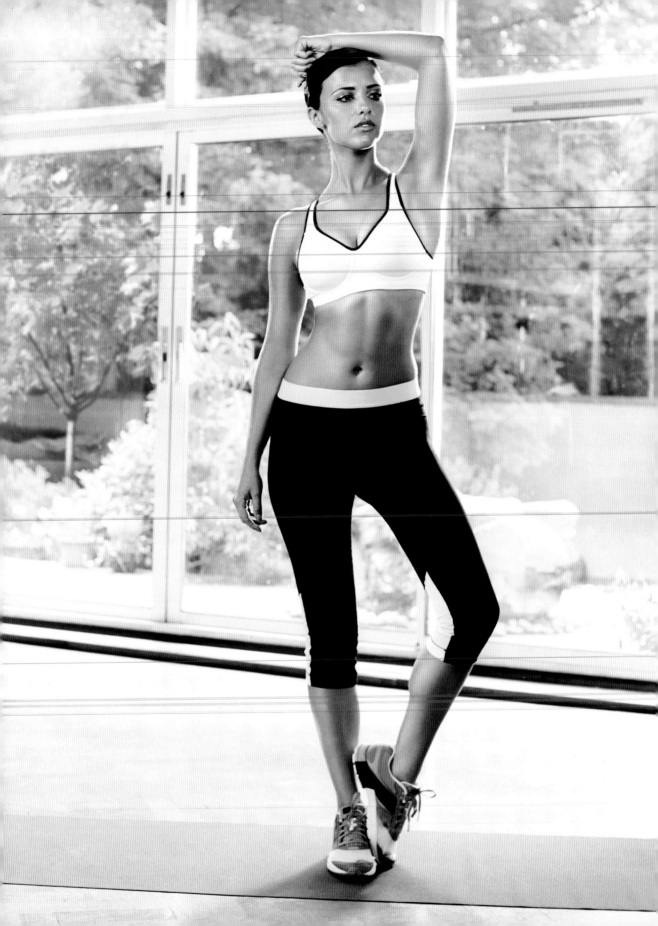

6

TRANSFORM

THE SIX-WEEK CHALLENGE

Now, here's what you've been waiting for: the six-week exercise and diet challenge. This isn't going to be easy BUT it will be worth it. Believe me. The plan is simple and easy to follow and you'll be able to incorporate it into your life easily. Excuses are not an option! The diet steps are given in chapter 3 (pages 78–107) but this is where you'll find the training programme.

Before you start it's really important to warm up...

Warming up is important for a number of different reasons but mainly so that you don't pull or tear any muscles and cause yourself an injury. The last thing you need when starting to exercise is an injury. It'll stop you before you even start. A warm-up will increase your heart rate as well as increasing blood circulation to your muscles, which will prepare you for your exercise routine. Your body temperature will rise and you'll be able to cope with a harder workout.

After warming up, you should focus on stretching your muscles which will also strengthen them.

REMEMBER to drink plenty of water before you start the workout as well as during.

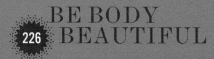

WEEK 1

This corresponds to the 'Cutting the C*@p' week for your diet (pages 78–85). Repeat the following training routine three times during this week (i.e. every other day).

1. SQUATS

Muscles used: quads (the fronts of your thighs) and glutes (your butt cheeks)

How to do it:

Stand with your feet hip-to-shoulder width apart, toes facing forwards,

Hands clasped together in front of your chest.

Bend your knees and push your bottom back as if you are trying to sit on a chair behind you.

Keep your chest up and your back straight.

Breathe in as you lower yourself, aiming to get your thighs parallel to the ground.

Breathe out, squeeze your thighs and glutes to return to standing.

Make sure your knees are straight and your hips are pushed slightly forwards in the standing position.

COMPLETE 10 REPS.

2. HIGH KNEES ON THE SPOT

Cardio (cardiovascular exercise raises your heart rate and, in turn, makes your metabolism move faster)

How to do it:

Stand with your feet hip width apart,

Chest up,

Belly button pulled in,

Shoulders back.

Bend your elbows to ninety degrees with your palms facing down.

Jogging on the spot, lift your knees up high so they touch your hands.

Stay up on your toes throughout for maximum effect.

CONTINUE FOR 30 SECONDS.

3. REVERSE LUNGES

Muscles used: quads and abs (between your belly button and your boobs)

How to do it:

Stand with your feet hip width apart,

Arms by your sides,

Chest up,

Belly button pulled in.

Take a large step backwards with your left foot.

Bend both knees,

Pushing your right knee over your toes

 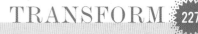

and lowering your left knee to just above the floor.

At the same time breathe in and lift your arms high above and slightly behind your head.

Stretch your ribs away from your pelvis.

Keep your chin parallel to the floor.

Return to your start position and change leg.

COMPLETE 10 REPS.

4. SQUAT JUMPS

Cardio; muscles used: quads

How to do it:

Stand with your feet together,

Belly button pulled in,

Chest up,

Shoulders back,

Hands clasped together in front of your chest.

Jump your feet wide to 1½ times shoulder width apart.

As your feet land, drop into a SQUAT position.

When your thighs reach parallel to the floor jump back to your start position.

COMPLETE 10 REPS.

5. PRESS-UPS

Muscles used: chest (the muscle above your boobs – chest exercises are good for lifting your boobs) and triceps (these are your bingo wings!)

How to do it:

Place your hands 1½ times shoulder width apart,

Fingers pointing forwards,

Knees and feet together,

Knees on the floor.

Keeping your hips up, make as straight a line as possible from hips to shoulders.

Keep your belly button pulled in.

Breathe in as you bend your elbows flaring them out to the side.

Do not allow your head to sag,

Keep your neck in line with your spine.

As you lower yourself down, try to make a triangle pattern with your hands and forehead.

You should not finish with your head in line with your hands.

With your back nice and straight, squeeze your chest and the backs of your arms.

Breathe out as you return to your start position.

COMPLETE 10 REPS.

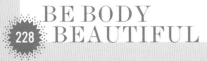

6. PLANK

Muscles used: abs, shoulders and back

How to do it:

Lying face down, place your elbows directly under your shoulders.

Keep your feet and knees together with the weight on your toes.

Lift your hips in line with your shoulders, creating a tabletop back.

(You should be able to rest your favourite drink without spilling a drop.)

Keep your belly button pulled in tightly, making your waist as small as possible.

Don't allow your head to drop down, make sure it is in alignment with your spine.

HOLD FOR 15 SECONDS.

Cool down

It's important not to forget to cool your body down after your workouts. It's just as important as warming up and again, stretching is key here. Light cardio is a great way of bringing your heart rate down. There's nothing worse for your body than doing a hard workout and then suddenly stopping. Your body goes into a kind of shock. Once your body is cooler, start to stretch the muscles out which will help relax them and increase circulation. PLEASE keep drinking water after you have finished so your body doesn't become dehydrated and REMEMBER to eat. You have just put your body through a tough workout so it needs food! Foods that are high in protein as well as carbs are great after a workout to bring back some of the energy you have just got rid of!

 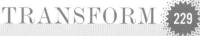

WEEK 2

This can be the week you feel like throwing the towel in. You should ache a bit and probably feel a bit tired. Please don't give up. This week is a turning point because your body is waking up to the changes you are trying to initiate. In terms of your diet, it corresponds to the 'Add More Antioxidants' week (pages 86–92). Repeat the following training routine three times during this week (i.e. every other day).

1. SQUATS

Muscles used: quads and glutes

See page 227 for instructions.

COMPLETE 15 REPS.

2. HIGH HEELS ON THE SPOT

Cardio; Muscles used: hamstrings (the backs of your legs)

How to do it:

Stand with your feet hip width apart,

Chest up,

Belly button pulled in,

Shoulders back.

Place your hands behind you,

Palms facing back just behind your bottom.

Jogging on the spot, kick your heels up behind you so they touch your hands.

Stay up on your toes throughout for maximum effect.

CONTINUE FOR 30 SECONDS.

3. ALTERNATE LUNGES

Muscles used: quads, glutes

How to do it:

Stand with your feet together,

Hands on hips.

Take a large step forwards with your right leg.

Bend both knees so you lower yourself to the ground.

Your back knee should not quite touch the floor.

Keep your chest up and shoulders back.

From here return to your start position and repeat on your other leg.

COMPLETE 15 REPS.

4. SQUAT JUMPS

Cardio; Muscles used: quads

See page 228 for instructions.

COMPLETE 10 REPS.

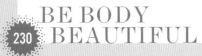

5. CRUNCHES

Muscles used: abs

How to do it:

Lying on your back,

Knees bent,

Feet flat,

Hands by your temples,

Elbows out,

Squeeze your abs and lift your upper back off the floor.

Breathe out as you lift, pulling your belly button down.

Keep a gap between your chin and your chest.

Breathe in as you return to the floor.

COMPLETE 15 REPS.

6. PRESS-UPS

Muscles used: chest and triceps

See page 228 for instructions.

COMPLETE 15 REPS.

7. OBLIQUE CRUNCHES

Muscles used: obliques (the muscles at the sides of your tummy – they accentuate your waistline and give you definition)

How to do it:

Lie on your back with your knees bent and together,

Feet flat on the floor.

Drop your knees to one side,

Hands by your temples.

Breathe out as you crunch your abs, lifting your upper back off the floor.

Keep a gap between your chin and your chest.

Pull your belly button down towards your spine.

Breathe in as you lower your body down.

COMPLETE 15 REPS WITH YOUR KNEES TO EACH SIDE.

8. PLANK

Muscles used: abs, shoulders and back

See page 229 for instructions.

HOLD FOR 30 SECONDS.

 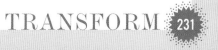

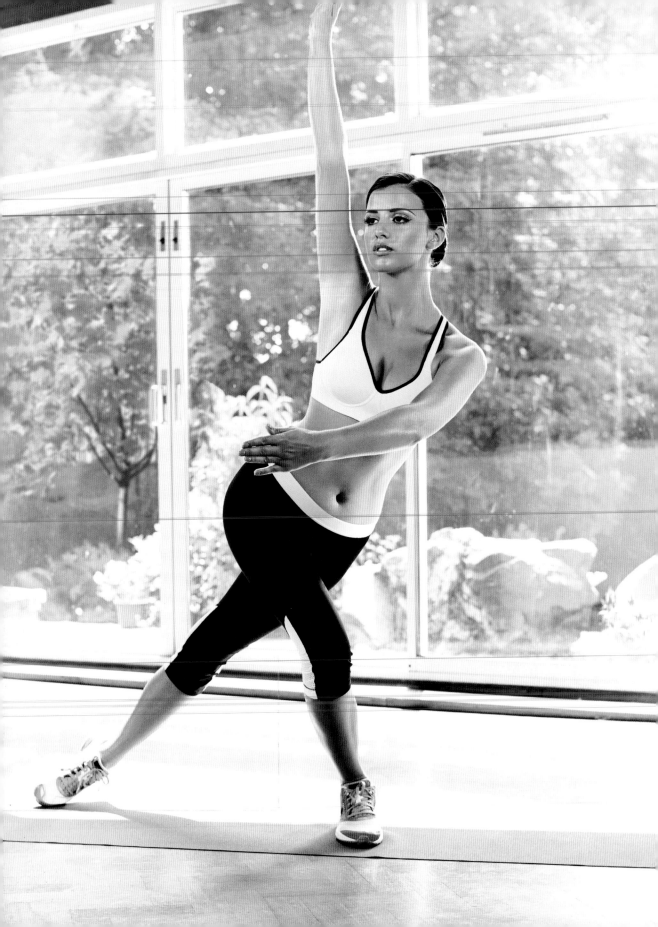

WEEK 3

By the end of this week you'll be halfway through the six-week challenge. Focus on that and it will get you through the week. You've come this far – don't stop now. In terms of the diet part of the challenge, you're now in the 'Wobble Wipeout' week (pages 93–4). Repeat the following training routine twice a day, every other day this week (i.e. six times in total).

1. SQUATS

Muscles used: quads and glutes

See page 227 for instructions.

COMPLETE 20 REPS.

2. ALTERNATE LUNGES

Muscles used: quads

See page 230 for instructions.

COMPLETE 20 REPS.

3. REVERSE LUNGES

Muscles used: quads and abs

See page 227 for instructions.

COMPLETE 20 REPS.

4. SQUAT INTO JUMPING JACKS

Cardio; Muscles used: quads and calves

How to do it:

Start standing with your feet together.

Squat down,

Keeping your knees and feet together.

Keep your back nice and straight,

Chest up,

Hands clasped in front of you at chest height.

From here jump up spreading your legs,

Land with your feet about 1½ times shoulder width apart.

At the same time, raise your arms straight out to the side.

Keeping your belly button pulled in,

Head up,

Jump back to the start position.

CONTINUE FOR 30 SECONDS.

5. PRESS-UPS

Muscles used: chest and triceps

See page 228 for instructions.

COMPLETE 20 REPS.

 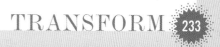

6. SIDE PLANK

Muscles used: obliques

How to do it:

Lying on one side,

Bend your elbow and place it directly underneath your shoulder.

Keep your body in a straight line,

One leg on top of the other,

Feet together,

Hips raised, so your torso is parallel to the ground.

Lift your top arm straight up in the air.

Don't let your head drop, keep the neck in line with your spine.

HOLD FOR 30 SECONDS AND HOLD THE OTHER SIDE FOR ANOTHER 30 SECONDS.

7. PLANK WITH TRAVEL

Muscles used: abs

How to do it:

Lying face down, place your elbows directly under your shoulders.

Keep your feet and knees together with the weight on your toes.

Lift your hips in line with your shoulders, creating a tabletop back.

Keep your belly button pulled in tightly, making your waist as small as possible.

Don't allow your head to drop down, make sure it is in alignment with your spine.

Shuffle to your right 3–4 times,

Then shuffle back to your left.

Keep your hips up to maintain your tabletop back position.

CONTINUE FOR 30 SECONDS.

8. CRUNCH WITH LEGS RAISED

Muscles used: abs

How to do it:

Lie on your back.

Lift your legs into the air pointing your toes to the ceiling.

Breathe out as you squeeze your belly button down towards your spine,

Crunching your abs to lift your upper back off the floor and reach your hands towards your toes.

Keep a gap between your chin and chest.

Breathe in as you lower your body back down.

COMPLETE 20 REPS.

9. LEG RAISES

Muscles used: lower abs (the muscles below your belly button, often referred to as a muffin top!)

Lying on your back with your arms by your sides,

Lift your legs into the air pointing your toes to the ceiling.

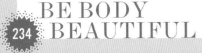

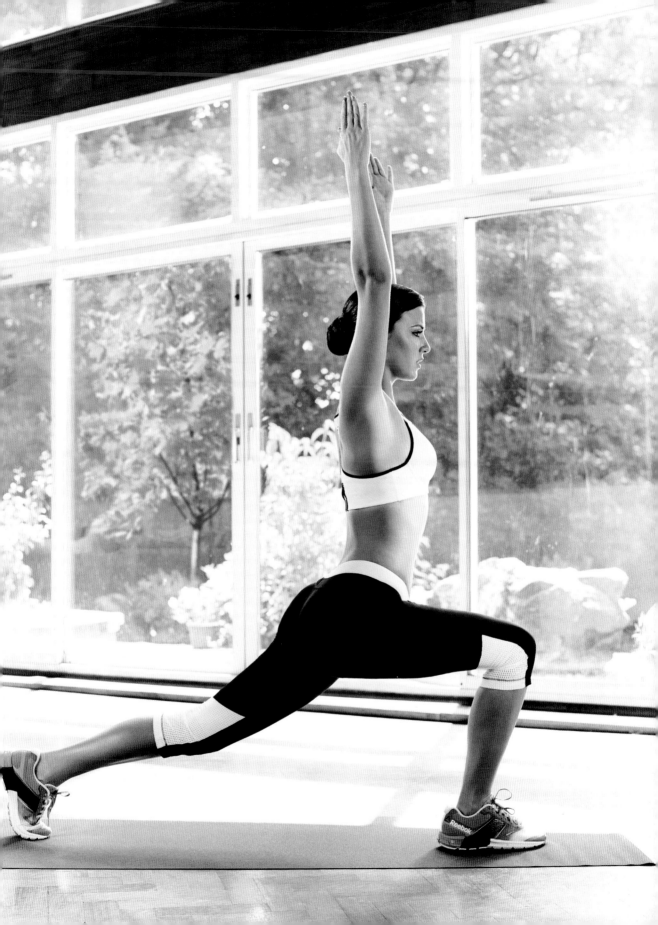

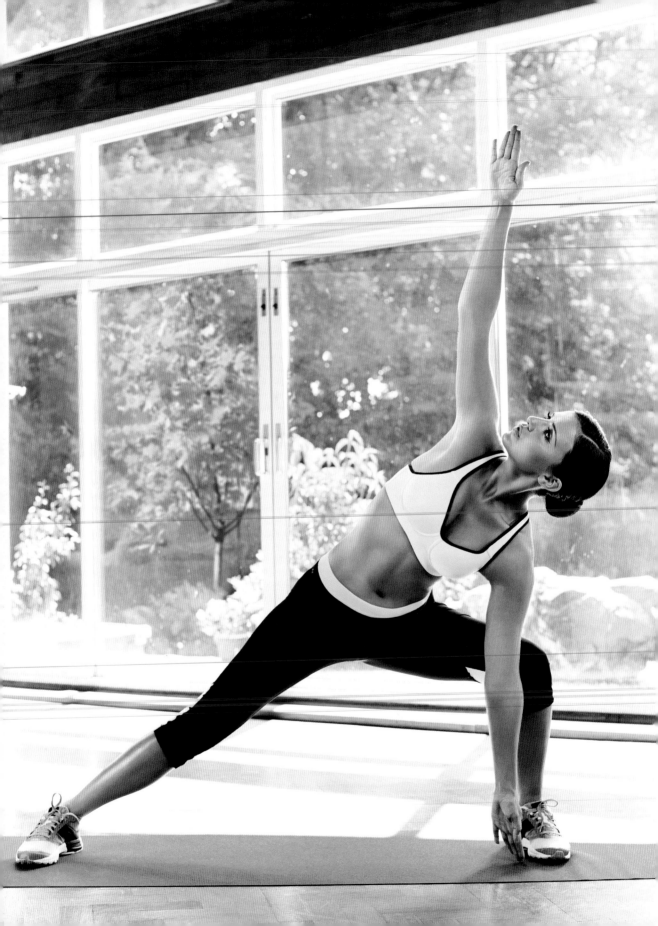

Keeping your legs straight, lower them towards the floor.

Ensure your lower back doesn't arch and remains in contact with the floor.

If you feel your lower back start to arch, stop lowering your legs and return to the start position.

Keep your belly button pulled in towards your spine at all times.

COMPLETE 10 REPS.

10. OBLIQUE CRUNCHES

Muscles used: obliques

See page 231 for instructions.

REPEAT 10 TIMES ON EACH SIDE.

WEEK 4

Come on – you're nearly there! After this there are only two more weeks and you'll have achieved so much. One final push. On the diet front, this is the 'Sup'ed Up' week (pages 96–8). Repeat the week 3 training routine but add 5 more reps to the counted exercises and 10 more seconds to the timed exercises. Remember you need to work out twice a day, every other day this week (i.e. six times in total).

WEEK 5

Feeling sore? You need to work through it and push yourself more this week than you have done so far. Some of the exercises should be becoming easier but parts of your body will be aching. Don't be put off. This means it's working. Your diet challenge is now heading into the 'Skin Food' week (pages 99 – 101). Repeat the following training routine twice a day, every other day this week (i.e. six times in total).

1. SQUATS

Muscles used: quads and glutes

See page 227 for instructions.

COMPLETE 20 REPS.

2. ALTERNATE LUNGES

Muscles used: quads

See page 230 for instructions.

COMPLETE 20 REPS.

3. SKIPPING – ROPE OPTIONAL

Cardio

How to do it:

Holding a skipping rope,

Keeping your belly button pulled in,

Stand nice and tall.

Skip.

 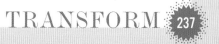

Jump over the rope as you turn it over your head and under your feet.

Stay on your toes for maximum effect.

CONTINUE FOR 40 SECONDS.

4. REVERSE LUNGES

Muscles used: quads and abs

See page 227 for instructions.

COMPLETE 20 REPS.

5. SQUAT INTO JUMPING JACKS

Cardio; Muscles used: quads and calves

See page 233 for instructions.

CONTINUE FOR 30 SECONDS.

6. PRESS-UPS

Muscles used: chest and triceps

See page 228 for instructions.

COMPLETE 20 REPS.

SIDE PLANK

Muscles used: obliques

See page 234 for instructions.

HOLD FOR 30 SECONDS AND THEN HOLD THE OTHER SIDE FOR 30 SECONDS.

N.B. You will need some dumbbells or any weight between 3–5 kg for the next few exercises ...

8. BENT-OVER ROW

Muscles used: upper back

How to do it:

Stand with your feet hip width apart.

Bend your knees,

Tilt forwards from your hips to approximately forty-five degrees.

Keep your belly button pulled in,

Spine straight.

Holding a dumbbell in each hand,

Let your arms hang straight down towards the ground,

Palms facing down.

Breathe out as you squeeze your shoulder blades together bending your elbows.

Bring the elbows out wide and towards the ceiling.

Breathe in as you return to the start position.

COMPLETE 15 REPS.

9. BICEP CURLS

Muscles used: biceps

How to do it:

Stand with your feet hip width apart,

Knees slightly bent,

Chest up,

Belly button pulled in,

Shoulders back,

Arms straight down by your sides.

Hold a dumbbell in each hand,

Palms facing up.

Breathe out as you squeeze your biceps to curl the weights up towards your shoulders.

Keep the elbows locked in mid air, they shouldn't move from your sides.

When your elbows are fully bent, breathe in and return the weights down by your sides.

COMPLETE 15 REPS.

10. UPRIGHT ROW

Muscles used: shoulders

How to do it:

Stand with your feet hip width apart,

Knees slightly bent,

Chest up,

Belly button pulled in,

Shoulders back,

Arms down in front of you.

Hold a dumbbell in each hand,

Palms facing down.

Bend your elbows up and out to the sides, raising them as high as possible.

The dumbbells should finish just under your chin.

Return to the start position.

COMPLETE 15 REPS.

11. BICEP AND SHOULDER COMBO

Muscles used: biceps and shoulders

How to do it:

Stand with your feet hip width apart,

Knees slightly bent,

Chest up,

Belly button pulled in,

Shoulders back,

Arms straight down by your sides.

Hold a dumbbell in each hand,

Palms facing up.

Breathe out as you squeeze your biceps to curl the weights up towards your shoulders.

When your elbows are fully bent, raise them out to the sides just like an UPRIGHT ROW.

From there, extend your arms so the weights are out in a LATERAL RAISE position, with your arms raised to shoulder height.

Lower the weights back down to the start position.

COMPLETE 15 REPS.

12. CRUNCH WITH LEGS RAISED

Muscles used: abs

See page 234 for instructions.

COMPLETE 20 REPS.

 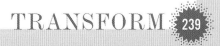

13. LEG RAISES

Muscles used: lower abs

See page 234 for instructions.

COMPLETE 10 REPS.

14. OBLIQUE CRUNCHES

Muscles used: obliques

See page 231 for instructions.

COMPLETE 10 ON EACH SIDE.

15. PLANK WITH HOPS

Muscles used: abs

How to do it:

Start in PLANK position.

(Lying face down, place your hands directly under your shoulders and push your upper body up.

Keep your feet and knees together with the weight on your toes.

Lift your hips in line with your shoulders, creating a tabletop back.

Keep your belly button pulled in tightly, making your waist as small as possible.

Don't allow your head to drop down, make sure it is in alignment with your spine.)

Jump your feet apart to just over shoulder width.

Keep your belly button pulled in and your hips in line with your shoulders.

Jump back to start position.

CONTINUE FOR 40 SECONDS.

16. MOUNTAIN CLIMBERS

Cardio

How to do it:

Start in PLANK position (variation 2).

(Lying face down, place your hands directly under your shoulders.

Keep your feet and knees together with the weight on your toes.

Lift your hips in line with your shoulders, creating a tabletop back.

Keep your belly button pulled in tightly, making your waist as small as possible.

Don't allow your head to drop down, make sure it is in alignment with your spine.)

Bring your right knee into your chest with a little hop.

Keep your left leg straight,

Keep your shoulders directly over your hands.

Hop again and swap your legs so that the left leg is bent and the right leg is straight.

Do not let your back sag,

Keep your belly button pulled in.

CONTINUE FOR 40 SECONDS.

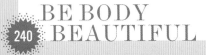

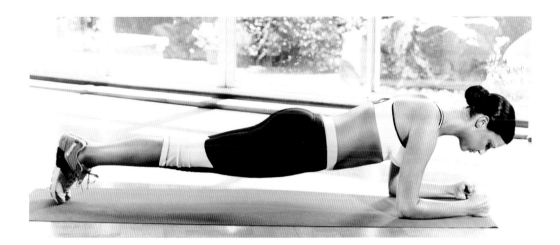

17. FROG PLANKS

Cardio

Start in PLANK position (variation 2).

(Lying face down, place your hands directly under your shoulders.

Keep your feet and knees together with the weight on your toes.

Lift your hips in line with your shoulders, creating a tabletop back.

Keep your belly button pulled in tightly, making your waist as small as possible.

Don't allow your head to drop down, make sure it is in alignment with your spine.)

Jump both feet to land flat, just outside of your hands.

From here, return to start position.

Do not let your back sag,

Keep your belly button pulled in.

CONTINUE FOR 30 SECONDS.

WEEK 6

It's the final push! You've got just one week left to go. Don't give in now. On the diet front, this is the 'Model Material' week (pages 103–6).

Repeat the week 5 training routine but increase how many times you do the routine as well as increasing the length of the workout to 1 hour.

⊃ ⊂ ▪ ⊂ ⊃ ⊂ ▪ ⊂ ⊃

So . . . How good do you feel now? Well done! You've done it. You've made it through the six-week challenge. You've made the changes your body needs. You will never look back. Guaranteed.

 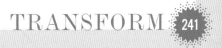

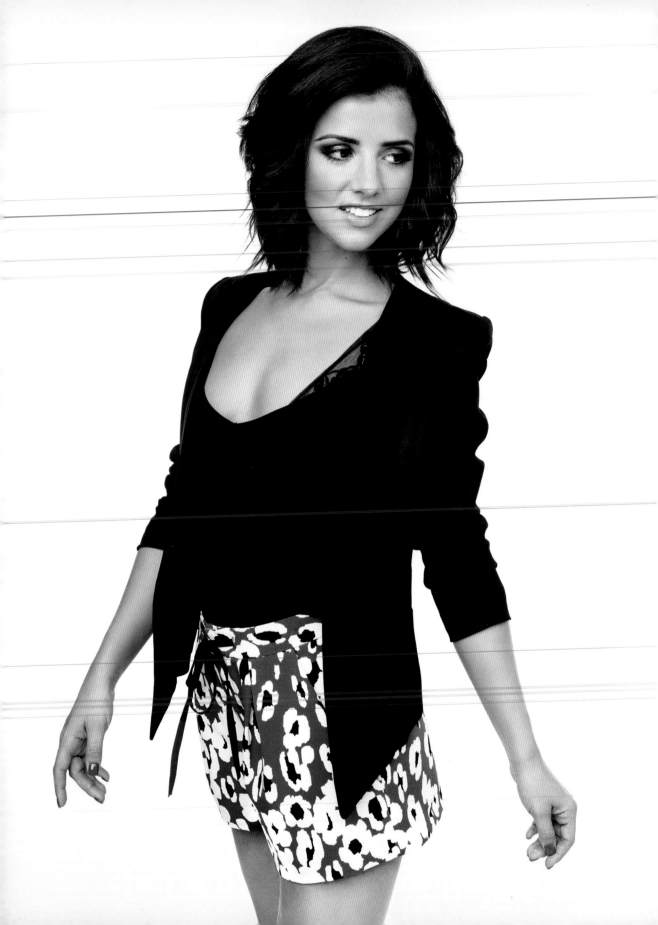

7

A HEALTHY, HAPPY NEW YOU

LOVE LIFE

When people think about my love life, I'm sure they straight away think of Mark Wright and Mario Falcone! I can't tell you how weird it is when suddenly other people are interested in who you are dating. It still seems surreal when I think about it now.

For a long time I haven't felt ready to get into a relationship, and that probably sums up the effect my last relationship had on me. But there is no point in dwelling on the past and the last two years have actually been both a steep learning curve and an opportunity to make things happen just for me, nothing to do with a guy. Girls, I really do believe that you need to be happy single in order to be happy in a relationship. Love yourself first before you fall in love with anyone else.

I was fourteen years old when I met my first boyfriend, Tommy, and we went out for four-and-a-half years. Tommy was a lovely guy but he found it hard to show me any real affection. I know I can be the same – showing affection isn't something that comes easily to me either – but when there are two of you like that it's not exactly the most compatible pairing. Tommy used to show his love in other ways, though. He'd spoil me and buy me presents and take me out for nice meals. Although he wouldn't cuddle me in public and I don't think he ever told me that he loved me. Not once. He was very loving towards his family, though, and he taught me a lot. Wherever he went he'd buy presents for his siblings. He was very caring; he just found it hard to show in any other way than through material objects. Tommy was quite old fashioned in a lot of ways. He wouldn't have anyone swear around me and he kept me very protected so, when we eventually split up when I was eighteen, life without him felt very strange. He was all I had known and suddenly I was alone, having to hit the social scene on my own and find my own way. It was weird.

At that stage I'd gone from being in a very long-term relationship, at a very young age, to being completely single and independent. Now that I'm older, hindsight and experience tell me that I was

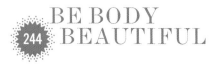

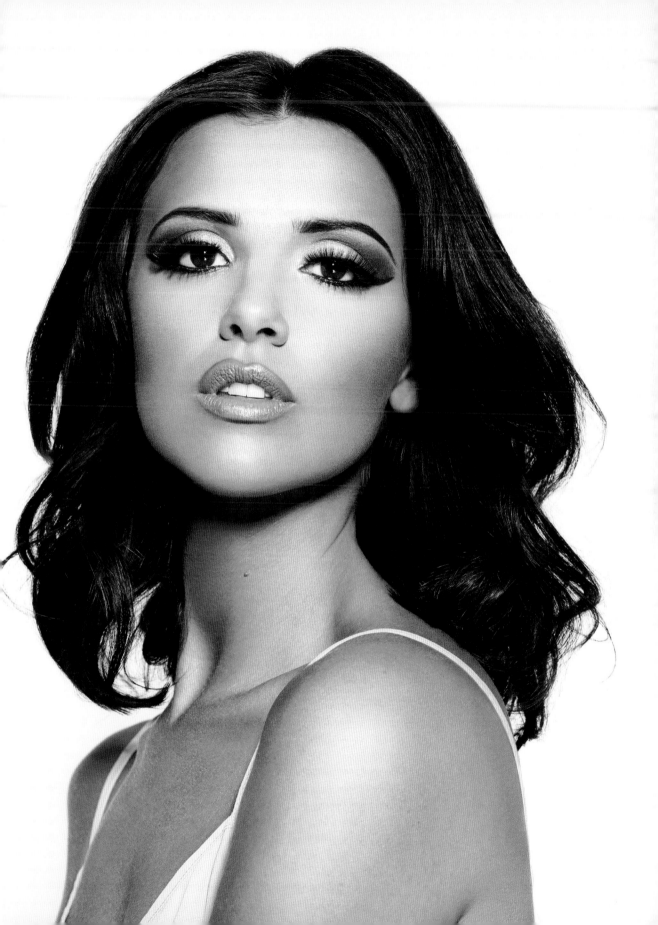

extremely young to be in such a relationship, but we are all brought up differently and I learned a lot. And in many ways I grew up more quickly, plus I didn't get into trouble or get hurt by a string of boys. So there are pros and cons.

Tommy had cheated on me and, although I took him back for a while, it didn't work out. Looking back, I can see that it couldn't have, after what had happened, but I was young and I was willing to give it another go. What you accept as a seventeen-year-old, you don't when you're in your twenties and thirties – and that's something only time can teach you. Would I take a guy back for cheating now? Absolutely not. But I thought I loved him when really I was probably just scared to be alone and scared to start all over again. We were so young that a break-up was inevitable.

Tommy was completely different to the men that I then started to hang around with after that. I met Mark Wright in Marbella, while I was still seeing Tommy. It was right at the end of our relationship but that's why nothing happened with Mark and when he asked me to have a drink with him that's all I had! I want to put a few things straight: I don't harbour any bad feelings about Mark Wright. It was a really simple situation. I was dating him and it ended up on telly for everyone to see and it all fell apart. Yes, there were bad times – I'm not going to lie. He did treat me awfully at times but now, with hindsight, having earned money for myself and with a successful business behind me, I can say, 'Fuck you.' What goes around comes around and I believe that.

⊙ • ⊕• •⊙ • ⊙• •⊕• •⊙

I was only nineteen years old when I started on *The Only Way Is Essex*: I was very young and I was incredibly naive. Ever since my introduction to the show there has been a spotlight on my physique. I was so nervous when I started – the producers had asked me to join a while back when I was working for the Forever Unique clothing company but I'd been worried about leaving my job for a reality show. I was concerned that the show would collapse and

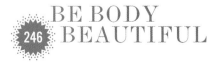

that I wouldn't have a job any more! Plus *TOWIE* didn't exactly pay the best – it wasn't great money and the hours were horrendous, but it did make me graft. I kept a paid job going through series one because I still wanted to be able to buy nice things and, as soon as I had enough money, I set up my first business – Lucy's Boutique.

On *TOWIE*, we'd sit about for hours waiting for our scenes to be filmed, very often in rooms with people that we hated or we used to date. It was awkward, but that atmosphere made for explosive television when we did finally get in front of the cameras. I would never say that I regret taking in part in *The Only Way Is Essex* because I don't. I am fully aware that I wouldn't be where I am now if it weren't for the show. But it's not a part of my life that I am proud of. It's like: I have got the box set but I'm not sure I'd want to open it. Of course people ask me whether I'd go back and you can never say never, but I am very happy right now. The concept was genius but, for me, playing out my life on television definitely affected me. I don't mean that negatively because, like I said, I wouldn't be where I am now if it wasn't for the show and I am incredibly grateful for all the opportunities it's given me, but when you go into a show like that you can't possibly know what you are letting yourself in for. It's impossible. And living your life in front of an audience can be difficult not only for you but also for your family. Seeing me all over national television crying my eyes out was hard for them. I think if my family was completely truthful, they would say that they were a bit embarrassed by the way I behaved on the show. They had no idea what was going to be on screen or what was happening or being filmed, and then they'd tune in and see me being mugged off and generally behaving completely out of character. My dad was watching his own daughter being messed about by some guy he'd never even met, knowing there wasn't anything he could do about it. That's embarrassing and I hated every minute of it. I used to try and stop them from watching the show. I'd come in and see Dad sitting in front of the TV and I'd go to my room. I could never watch it with

 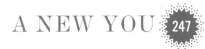

him. In the end I wanted to leave the show because I wanted to be proud of something and I wasn't proud of that.

I think people imagine that I must have been desperate to be a part of *TOWIE*, but really I was just a kid who had a TV company approach them to go on a show. What was I supposed to say? Most people being offered an opportunity like that aren't going to pass it up. I got swept along with something and into situations that in retrospect I never should have let myself get into. Like with Mark. I looked like a complete idiot a lot of the time. I played a part but for me it was my real life, my real emotions being played out for everyone to see. Looking back now, it's embarrassing. It wasn't until I left the show that I fully appreciated how much. I think because Tommy was the only guy I'd properly been out with and he was all that I knew, it lulled me into a false sense of security and then when Mario went on to treat me like he did I was a stupid blubbering wreck!

You can't underestimate how hard it is to have your real love life played out on television. I know I agreed to it, and it's not even something that I regret or wish I had done differently, but it's a part of my life I don't want to dwell on. I was humiliated for a lot of it and I don't think anyone got much of an impression of who I actually am. I spent most of my time on screen as some kind of victim or crying over the way I'd been treated. When, in reality, I couldn't be further from THAT person. Since *TOWIE*, it's been hard to try and change people's perceptions and, even now, I'm not sure I totally have because a lot of people's lasting memories of me are from my relationship with Mario. Some of the best and some of the worst times of my whole life were played out for everyone to see and I can never change that.

Mario and I went out for just under two years and he was a very special part of my life. For that reason and many more I don't want to lay into him. We had some very good times and some very, very bad times. But I owe him in part for the strength I have today because if I were back on *TOWIE* now I'd be a very different person. You certainly wouldn't see me breaking down every five seconds.

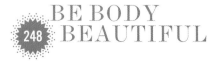

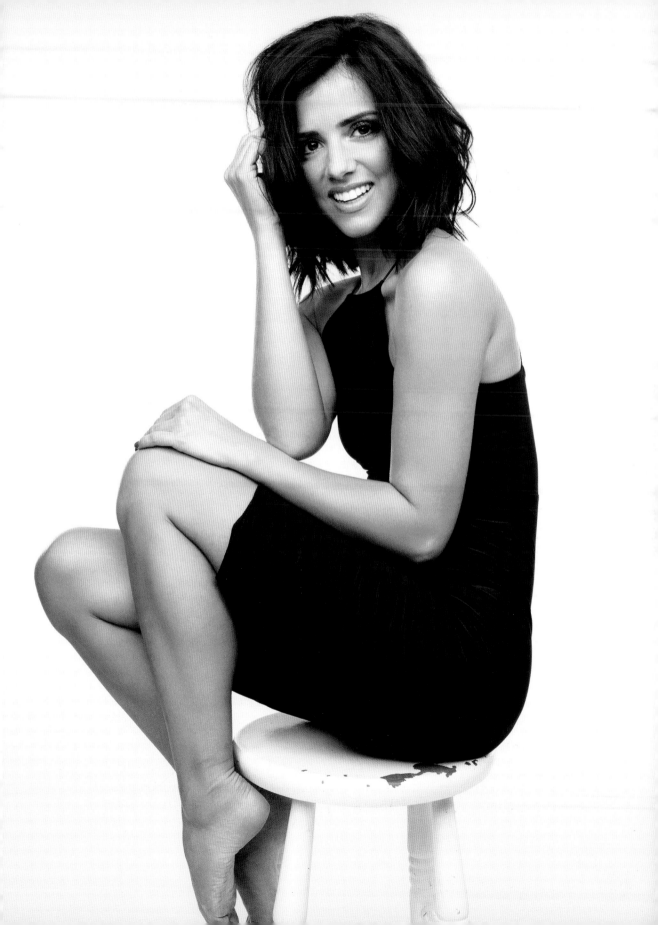

We had met long before I was on the show – Mario was after me when I was still with Tommy but I wasn't interested then. He chased me for ages, texting me and asking me if I was still with my boyfriend. At one time he used to ask Tommy in the gym if we were still together. It was bizarre, him chatting to my boyfriend to basically check if he could make a move on me! He was desperate to go out on a date but I'd heard he was a player and, besides, I was still seeing someone else.

Years later, after I had finished with Mark Wright, Mario got back in touch and then I was in a bar and I saw him. Something in my brain clicked and I said to the girls, 'He's quite hot actually!' I remember looking at him and thinking, 'He's pretty good-looking – why have I been turning him down all this time?' So I plucked up the courage and I went to go and speak to him but, as I got near him, he swung this girl around and kissed her right in front of me. I thought, 'Well, that's told me!' I'd turned this guy down for months but when I was ready he had moved on. I was so annoyed but it was my just desserts. I tried to style it out and walk back to where I had left my drink but it was so bloody obvious and I felt like a real idiot. My move on Mario had completely backfired! I drank up as quickly as I could and went home. That night I couldn't stop thinking about him and the fact he was now with someone else. The more I couldn't have him, the more I wanted him. I knew I had no right to him and that it had been me who had turned him down in the first place but that didn't help much when it was late at night and that was all I could think about! I didn't have to wait long though, because the next day I received a text from him saying that he had dumped his girlfriend for me and asking me to go out for a drink with him. Of course, I said yes! That was when I found out that Mario was a tailor and my opinion of him went up because most boys in Essex are arrogant traders and I totally assumed he was one of those. When I found out what he did for a living, I thought what an inspirational trade to have learned. The relationship moved pretty quickly. I think we were both infatuated. It had been so long coming that when we did

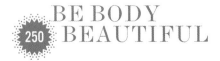

finally get together we moved in fast-forward! It wasn't long before we were spending every waking moment with each other. I hated being apart from him and I'd always be hoping that he'd text me from work because I missed him that much when we were apart. You know, that first flush of . . . I was going to say love but it was probably lust!

I would wait at Mario's house until he got home from work – we were like an old married couple in a lot of ways. It became a habit and routine very quickly but I loved it! It felt really normal and it was easy; I felt comfortable and loved. It was quite a while before Mario joined me on *TOWIE* and it was me, believe it or not, who talked him into joining the show. He was quite reluctant, which seems weird now because he loves being famous! The show's producers were on his case too. They were really keen to get him on once they knew we were dating. They'd met him a couple of times when he dropped me off on set and I think that they could see that he'd be a hit with the viewers, so they were trying to persuade him too! He was worried it would impact on his job and, like me, he was also worried that if it didn't work out with the television show then he would be left with nothing. I think he liked the idea of being a part of the show – like his heart said yes but his head was saying no. We talked about it a lot – going over the positives and negatives practically every night – and I really wanted him to be on *TOWIE* with me. In the end I convinced him and he agreed to come on the show. I made a monster of him, didn't I? So, in retrospect, it wasn't the best idea and it put a huge pressure on our relationship.

In the beginning things were fine, but the novelty of having him on set with me quickly wore off. It's like working with your partner in the same office and magnifying it 500,000 times because we were also being filmed for a reality television show! I could never have imagined that Mario coming on to the show would have such a detrimental effect on our relationship – if I had I would never have suggested it. The pressures of living out everything in front of the camera proved harder than anything and obviously there was Mark too – I had had a relationship with him and so there was

 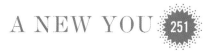

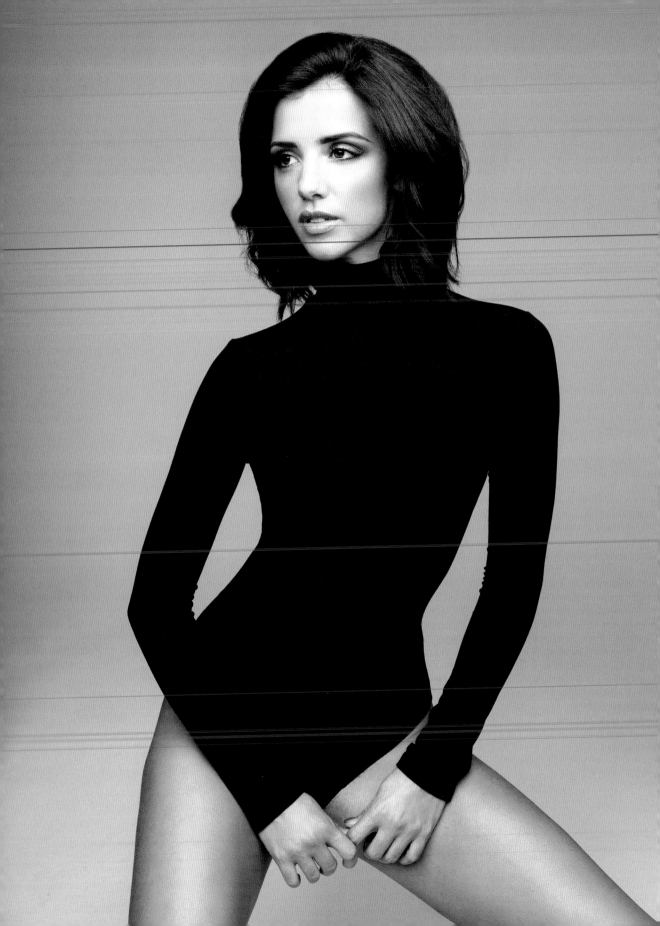

that whole dynamic, which at times could be awkward. I'm not a massively jealous person but everything gets distorted on a show like *TOWIE* and you start to behave out of character. It's weird and hard to explain but tiny things that I never would have thought twice about before were being blown completely out of proportion. Almost immediately Mario seemed very different to me. For some people, getting recognition in the street or some kind of notoriety can change them and I think it went to Mario's head a bit. He was getting a lot of attention and he was enjoying it. I could see that and it began to eat away at me. I started to worry that the flirtations would end up being more and, of course, I was right, they did.

Living in front of the camera began to take its toll on both of us. I don't think either of us knew what was genuine and, by the end, it all felt so fake. Mario would say one thing to me privately and then, on screen, do something else. It was exhausting and confusing and it was breaking down any self-esteem that I had. The experience was destructive and yet I was in the thick of it and I didn't seem to be able to get control of the situation. The line between reality and reality television became a big old blur to me and I think Mario had become suckered into another world, the famous world. Eventually it took him over completely, which I think is hugely dangerous. He needed someone to get hold of him and bring him back down to earth, but that wasn't going to be me – he was too far gone and any influence that I might have had over him had been eroded completely.

Unbelievably in all of that craziness – albeit when things hadn't got nearly as bad as they did in the end – Mario asked me to marry him and, of course, it was filmed! He had hired a private boat and we were being filmed for an *Only Way Is Marbs* special. He'd organized champagne and laid out rose petals. It was so romantic. He was a romantic guy and I loved that about him: he could be really thoughtful when he wanted to be. There's so much about that day that people don't know, it's hilarious. So, basically, he'd hired this boat and I'd been on it a bit before the proposal but I suffer very badly from seasickness and I started to feel really ill almost straight

 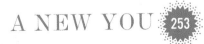

away. I kept asking to get off the boat and saying that I was going to be sick but obviously the plan was for him to ask me to marry him on the boat, so everyone was keen for me to try and stay on board. I hated every minute of it because I felt SO ILL. When I got back on I could see all the petals and champagne and something clicked in my head and I knew what was going to happen. I just had this feeling that he was going to pop the question. The boat felt really rocky and that whole scene, while we are sitting on the edge of the boat, I seriously thought that I was going to throw up. I mean, it probably is the most romantic thing anyone has ever done for me. He had had a ring made especially for me and it fitted perfectly and, in some ways, it was a dream come true. I was marrying the man that I loved and thought I wanted to spend the rest of my life with, and I thought us getting engaged would solve any problems we might have had – which, as it turned out, couldn't have been further from the truth. If you watch the clip you can see me keep putting my hand over my mouth. I'm saying, 'Oh my God, oh my God,' over and over again but really I was literally being sick in my mouth and swallowing it. How disgusting is that? Then I kissed him! I wanted to get off that boat so much. I felt so ill it was ridiculous. I still don't know to this day how I managed to stop myself actually puking all over Mario! There we were, trying to film this most romantic scene and I was being sick in my mouth. What no one realized either was that I had taken a load of seasickness tablets and then I started to drink, like a complete idiot. The combination of the tablets and the drink made things much worse. I was getting drunker by the second and when we went for a romantic meal after the proposal I passed out in my pasta. Mario had to carry me up to bed – I was a complete mess and I can tell you he got nothing that night! It's funny now but at the time it was a bit embarrassing.

∘ · ◈ · ∘ · ∘ · ◈ · ∘

Mario proposed to me in June 2012 and the following February, after we called off our engagement but were still dating, we went

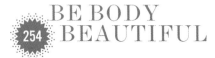

BE BODY
BEAUTIFUL

on a trip to Mexico. Things between us had taken a massive turn for the worse. All those words from Mario about never wanting to be with anyone else were complete rubbish and he had a wandering eye. All that time he'd tried to get me, he finally had me and he threw it away by sleeping with other girls.

I have never spoken openly about the reasons we split up. It was such a public relationship but there are parts of it that I feel should still remain private. Like with any couple there are things you don't want splashed everywhere. I'm only going to touch on the things in our relationship that relate to why I have become the person I am today. There are definite points that have made me stronger.

The holiday in Mexico was a key turning point for me. I knew deep down that things weren't right, but I didn't really want to address the problems. I wanted to stay in the bubble that I was in. I wanted to ignore all the stories saying that Mario had cheated on me and I wanted to believe him but, of course, I'm not stupid and those doubts inevitably started to affect me and, in turn, the relationship. I never, ever wanted to believe he had cheated on me and I think for any relationship to work you must have trust or it will fail. I didn't have any firm proof that he was cheating and until there was I didn't want to doubt him because in my mind that was unfair on him. He was promising me none of it was true and I, maybe foolishly, believed him. I didn't want to believe that he had done that to me. He had told me that he wanted to spend the rest of his life with me so I didn't want to throw all of that away on hearsay. Of course, when you become famous a lot of girls make stories up for money and fame and Mario had an explanation for each one. But inevitably it still niggled at me, as I think it would with anyone. Gradually the relationship started to slip and, in truth, by the end of it I was a bit of a mess.

We shared a house, we shared our dogs Bentley and Lola, and we had been engaged. Looking back now, I can see I was far, far too young to get engaged and I can honestly say that I would never get engaged on television again! It ruins it. A proposal should be the

 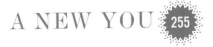

most special thing to happen to a girl; you grow up dreaming about it and it should be something between just the two of you. I can't bear to watch that clip of when he asked me – it is so horribly cheesy and awful. But I don't blame Mario for it. We were very much in love and we were having an amazing time. It is very easy at such a young age to get caught up in a moment and be bulldozed along with what you and everyone around you thinks would be right.

When we called off the engagement it was an instant relief. It was hard to get to that point and to make that decision. I wanted it to work out but I knew it couldn't. A relationship has to be built on trust and the trust had been wiped out from ours. My older self that now has more life experience tells me that it clearly wasn't right and back then even when I wasn't at my strongest and was quite confused I knew that marrying Mario would have been wrong on so many levels. There will always be a special place in my heart for Mario; I just wish that I had never introduced him to *TOWIE* and that he had stayed doing his job as a tailor. I was so proud of what he did and when things were good between us they were excellent. I know that Mario deeply regrets what happened between us and his behaviour at the time and, honestly, I wish him nothing but happiness now. I wouldn't have always been able to say that because my feelings were still tied up in it but now I just feel kind of sorry for him because he lost the girl he always wanted by doing something stupid. Fame blurred his vision and yet, as I told him so often, he's very talented and could have had an amazing career. He could have achieved big things without becoming famous but I think he became obsessed with fame and that was where we were fundamentally different. I was determined to start a business and build my life around that. It's a shame he hasn't stayed off *TOWIE* so he can start to rebuild the 'Mario' that I originally fell in love with. I think it would have been the best thing for him not to be on the show any more. He could have got back to being the kind and sensitive guy he once was because I do genuinely wish for him to be happy.

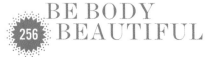

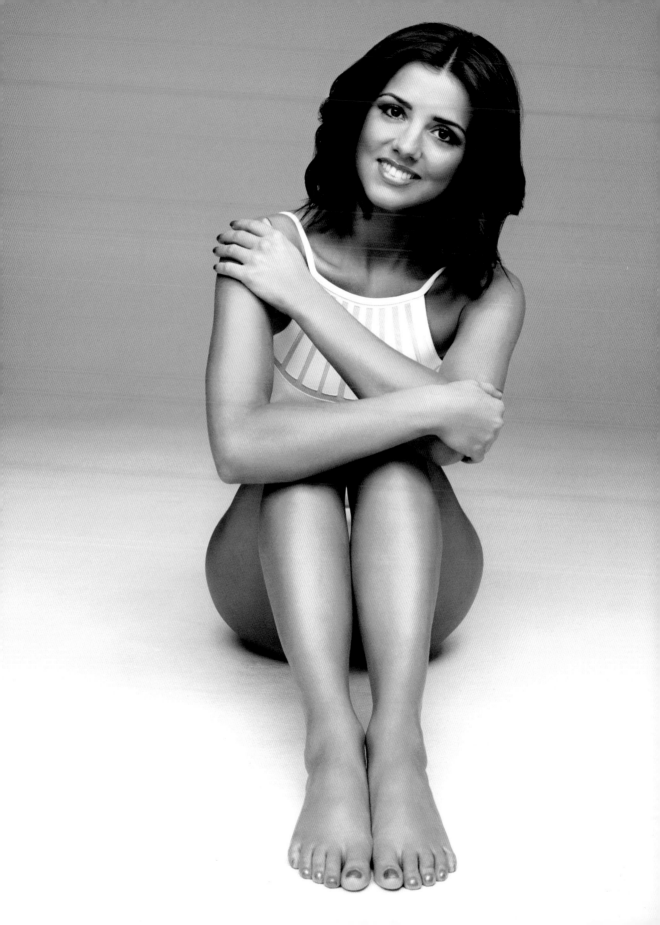

After my relationship with Mario ended I threw myself into work – that's my defence mechanism! My agent, Scarlett, kept me busy and cheered me up with lots of lovely opportunities. It's weird because at the time it was really difficult but I was also in awe of all the things I was then able to do that I'd never thought possible. That's not to say it was because of no longer being with Mario – it absolutely wasn't – but I think it's important for any young girl or boy to appreciate that if you are in an intense, committed relationship very young then you inevitably hold back from doing things just for yourself. Sometimes you can't have it all and I felt like this was my time to shine.

I think it's fair to say that on *TOWIE* our audience respected me for not accepting being treated badly and I took that same mentality with me when it came to my work. I guess I did a lot of growing up throughout that time too, and I definitely started to get more and more into fashion. We did some really cool shoots abroad and started working with big brands. We approached every project with real passion, as if we wanted to make it stand out and be cool and different. When my agent suggested I sign with a modelling agency it was as if she was having a laugh! Then, in a weird twist of fate, my agent received a call from a couple of agencies saying they'd seen a shoot of me they loved and everything just fell into place.

I remember going into the offices of Select model management and just knowing right then they were the ones for me. We met with a few different agencies and each had their different benefits but Select was so cool I could not actually believe that they, the biggest model agency in the world, were willing to sign me, Lucy from Essex, who has curves and is five foot six! But they did and I can honestly say it's been a blast. From catwalk shows and fronting international advertising campaigns to hilarious trips all over the world with my modelling agent, Kirsty, and Scarlett. I still have to pinch myself.

Sometimes, girls, things are worth the wait. I can't tell you how grateful I am to the team I have around me that helped make that happen.

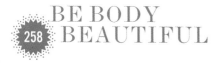

Dating Tips

After all of my experiences in love I think I have come to understand the first rule of love: there are no rules! Every relationship is unique and what makes one can break another. But at the ripe old age of twenty-three, I have had my fair share of experiences and I think that I have learned quite a lot about men. The biggest piece of advice of all is that you don't need a man to be happy. However, the sooner you are happy and comfortable in yourself, the sooner you will be attractive to a man. Of that I am sure. Still, there are some things I try to remember when I'm on the lookout for a new guy, or if I've just started something with someone special.

First and foremost, you can throw all of the old-fashioned advice out of the window. Don't worry about waiting for a guy to come to you. They're not mind readers so they won't know if you're interested in them unless you say so or make it very obvious! Subtlety isn't their greatest strength, is it? Of course, throwing yourself at someone isn't the best idea either, but it's totally cool to approach a guy if you fancy him. Most guys worth having will find that confidence attractive and sexy. Men enjoy the thrill of the chase and if a man is into you he will chase you. Enjoy it – it's often the best part. Every girl is desperate to have those butterfly 'first-flush-of-love' feelings and they start when the guy you fancy decides to make his move. This part always goes too quickly so make the most of it.

Pretending to be someone else is always a let-down for the other side because inevitably the 'real' you will come out! The key here is to relax and be yourself and soon enough someone will love you for it. This obviously isn't a ticket to give up washing and to wear your onesie that you secretly love every day, but if you keep all of your actions within the confines of 'normal', it should do the trick and have the desired effect on the one you're after. Look after yourself like you should do anyway. Waxing maintenance, that sort of thing – you know what I'm talking about. Don't just do it for a bloke, do it because you want to feel good about yourself.

 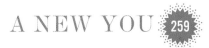

I hate guys who play games. I've got so many friends who waste loads of time trying to interpret the weird messages guys send them. Like, one guy my friend was seeing seemed to really like going out with her, but as soon as he left he wouldn't reply to her texts for days. It was total mixed messages and hard for her to know where she stood. When she finally cracked and confronted him, after he went for a week without speaking to her and then suddenly texted saying he had only just charged his phone (I know, what a rubbish excuse), he just said that he wasn't looking for a girlfriend and wanted to keep things casual. She carried on letting him treat her like that because she was really into him and secretly she probably thought she could change his mind but in reality that was never going to happen. We could all see how stressed the situation was making her – never knowing where he was or if he was seeing other girls. Thankfully in the end, and with a lot of encouragement from her mates, she saw sense and decided to sack him off. Not a moment too soon in my book. If it works for you and you only want something casual then that's fine but as soon as your emotions start to get involved bin a guy who plays games.

Don't stand for someone messing you around. I have done it on too many occasions – giving boys the benefit of the doubt – but, seriously, it never comes good. I have the scars to show! I know it's hard to dump someone if you really like them, but there's no point being with a person who doesn't recognize or appreciate how great you are. If they don't feel the same way about you or don't treat you well at the beginning then it can only ever get worse. People don't change overnight. There are so many good guys out there – don't let one loser stop you from finding them.

Single girls will know that the worst paradox of love is that it rarely rears its head when you look for it. I don't know why this is, but when I go out hoping to meet someone, I never do. But if I'm on a girl's night out just having fun with my friends and not thinking about men, chances are that's when I'll meet someone special. So if you're single, just try to concentrate on the things you like doing and someone will

BE BODY
BEAUTIFUL

come along when you least expect it. Don't forget: LOVE yourself.

Once you're in a relationship, it's very tempting to spend every moment together, but, as I learned from moving in too quickly in the past, you end up going at a hundred miles an hour. Rushing to push your relationship up to the next notch isn't, in my opinion, the best idea. The honeymoon period's the best bit, right? So why try and get it over with as soon as possible? I always get sucked into wanting to spend all of my time with that one person. It's very easy to slip into being that person who sacks all their friends off as soon as they get a boyfriend – I bet we all know someone who has done that and I've probably been guilty of it too in the past. After all, that's the natural reaction when you're in love. You just need to step back and take a few minutes to remember it! No matter how much you love your new boyfriend, you'll never be able to rely on him as much as you can rely on your friends.

You shouldn't spend all of your time stopping yourself from hanging out with your new guy – you do need to get to know each other – but remember to keep being you. Don't spend every night at their place and make sure you have a few nights apart each week to keep things fresh. It's really tempting to move in with each other quickly. You don't have to waste all of that time travelling, right? And you get to be with the guy you are totally infatuated with – what could go wrong? There's no right time to make the move and the right time to live together varies from couple to couple, but waiting until you know him really well can only up the chances of it working. You'll already know all of each other's little foibles so there are no nasty surprises.

Keeping a bit of mystery in the relationship is also key to keeping the spark alight. There's always a point with a new boyfriend where you can get too comfortable around him. And while no good guy is going to pack his bags the moment he sees you shaving your legs, it's nice to keep some things private. Mystery is the main component of eroticism. Of course you can't spend every night pretending you're strangers, but holding a few things back is no bad thing.

 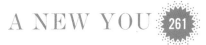

CONFIDENCE

You'll know by now that I've had my low moments, the same as everyone else. I've had my heart broken but I've learned how to bounce back and enjoy life again. I can't stress enough how important it is to be happy and single before you even try to embark on a relationship. It's imperative.

As any girl who's come out of a relationship knows, it wrecks your confidence and it takes a long time to heal yourself before you feel like someone else could love you again.

There are lots of ways to build up your self-esteem and start to feel yourself, though. I threw myself into training. It took my mind off thinking about what had happened and it kept me busy. There's a lot of time when you break up with someone that isn't accounted for any more and you need to fill that with something or else you start to go backwards, remembering all the good times rather than the reality of what the relationship had become. For me, aside from exercise, friends were the best medicine and they picked me up and really helped to get me through those initial weeks. As the saying goes, time is a great healer and the less you are with someone, the less you want to be and the happier you become. Turning to exercise was a great thing for me because it started to make me feel better about myself. The better I looked, the more he probably wished he hadn't messed up as badly and that helped in a way too. It gave me a new confidence and was part of the healing process. Turning to comfort food and putting on weight won't help anyone in this situation. Guaranteed. You will feel more sluggish, you won't want to go out and your skin will become spotty. This will NOT help you give the two-finger salute to your ex! I'm not advocating revenge but it's very sweet when your ex sees you walking down the road looking better than you did when you were with them . . .

It's very hard to cope when one moment you have everything you've ever wanted – a house, a relationship, a cute little puppy and a future

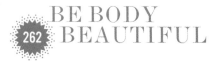

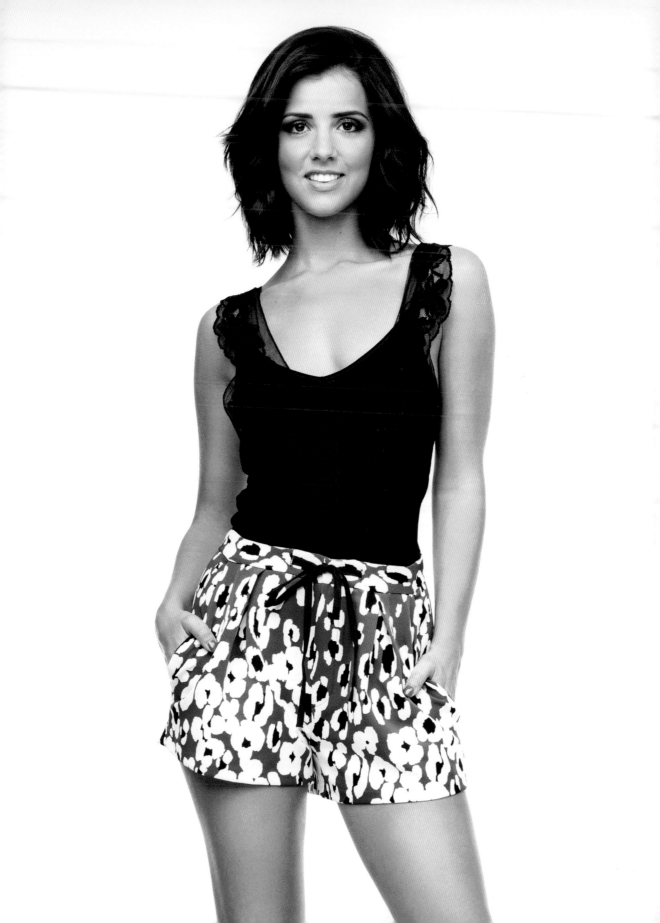

– and then it's ripped away when you're least expecting it. To be fair, I was the one who called it quits with Mario, but that never makes it any easier. I felt I had no choice but to tear us apart. No matter how upset it made me feel, I knew staying together would make me more unhappy in the long run. I just kept that thought in my head whenever I was near breaking point and that helped me get through some of those lonely nights.

Maybe the worst thing about that particular break-up was that it was conducted so publicly and I had to read everything that was being written. So many lies and so many things that were completely untrue! I never wanted to tell my side, though – I still don't and I've always kept a dignified silence on some of the major relationships I've had.

Not only was the press having a field day, Mario and I were also still filming for *TOWIE*. I'd have to watch him getting it on with other girls while I was still feeling massively raw about it all. Watching Mario flirt with other women on screen was pretty tough to watch. It's like when you see your ex getting with someone else in a nightclub, but there's no chance of a quick taxi home and consolatory chat with your best mate. Your heartbreak is there whenever you turn on the telly, go on the Internet or pick up a newspaper or magazine. It was hard but I just learnt to deal with it and I think I'm now a much stronger person because I've gone through the pain. In the end, I guess, you've got to learn the hard way. Now I know how to put myself first and not sacrifice my happiness for anyone.

๑ · ๑ · ๑ · ๑ · ๑ · ๑

How to Paint a Brave Face on it All

It's really easy to feel negative about how you look when your relationship isn't working. When my engagement ended, I turned all of my stress on my body, punishing it with tough workouts. Like I've mentioned I did go off my food and I did lose a lot of weight. I'd forget to eat regularly but I think that's quite normal. To try to block

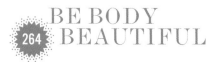

out how rubbish the end of the relationship was making me feel, I lost myself in exercise – it became my passion and my addiction. Although I couldn't control what had happened to my relationship, I could call the shots when it came to my workouts. I also started to really enjoy doing them and I genuinely forgot about all of my worries.

Training got my endorphins pumping and gave me something to focus on at a time when everything else was falling apart. Hands down, I'd say it's the best cure for a broken heart. After all, as I've already pointed out, there's nothing better than bumping into an ex and showing off your new killer body. But don't forget, if you're exercising to boost your confidence remember to keep up your food intake – something I admit I did let slip. Eat healthy food, but make sure you are eating enough to sustain your workouts. The more you do, the more protein you will need in your diet. Cutting out refined sugars also really helped me because suddenly I realized I didn't really need them. (SO MANY people don't even realize that something they are eating, which they may think is healthy, will have a whole heap of sugar in it.) It's particularly important to eat well when you start a new training regime, otherwise you'll feel tired and crabby all of the time, which is counterproductive, especially if you are at a low point in your life anyway. This is something I really had to take on board during my training for *Tumble*, when I was often working out for five hours a day. If I didn't eat enough food, I'd be a complete monster and I'd never have achieved that level of training on a daily basis.

I've said it before and I'll say it again: I do recognize that I went through a time of being too thin and it was a mixture of a few things including the anxiety of my break-up. I was eight stone back then, but now I weigh eight stone ten pounds and I think that that's a very healthy weight for me. All the training for *Tumble* made me feel strong, and strength in fitness is something that a lot of women strive to achieve. My body has definition and I feel confident and amazing. It's an incredible way to feel.

 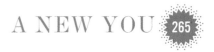

How Lucy has Built up her Self-esteem

However healthily you're eating and exercising, though, it's still very important to remember not to be too hard on yourself. If you have a naughty day and want to indulge in a pizza, let yourself. What I try and do to keep myself on track is be good during the week and then relax a bit on the weekend. So I'll save myself some treats to have on a Friday night like a Bellini cocktail or a piece of chocolate cake or some bread. (I haven't bought a loaf of bread since I've been in my flat!) I think this is a great way of motivating yourself during the week – you can push through being healthy for five days with the prospect of a gooey pudding at the end! You don't want to become the person who feels guilty about everything you eat. Life is for living and that's a horrible way to be. If you think this way you will always have a goal and your healthy eating far outweighs those naughty moments. You don't want to be the one in a restaurant ordering a chicken Caesar salad without dressing and without croutons – it's dull and it's starving your body of some of the pleasures in life that it should be allowed to indulge in on occasion. It's very easy for your weight and diet to become an obsession, and this is a great way of not letting that happen. You know you're still going to look great, so you can enjoy your treats guilt-free.

On a similar note, the most important way to keep yourself happy – beyond exercise or healthy eating or working on your career – is by loving yourself. When I was a teenager, I went through moments of not feeling very confident – like most teenagers do. At that age you only need one person to knock you and then you start questioning everything from what you're wearing to what you're saying. My mum always used to say to me that confidence is attractive in a person and to believe in myself. It's not always that easy but if you can focus on that then her advice is so true.

So, I guess what I'm trying to say is learn to love yourself. It's a phrase that's used again and again, but it's true: If you don't accept yourself, no one else will.

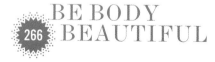

MY TOP TEN CONFIDENCE TIPS

1 Be yourself. It can be easy to pretend you're someone you're not when you're trying to impress a new group of friends or a guy. But you're most attractive when you're being who you really are.

2 Surround yourself with friends who make you feel good about who you are. Don't let other people's negativity make you feel bad. It's draining and it's unhealthy. There are a lot of people who can be jealous. Don't let them get you down – it's their insecurity. Not yours.

3 Work out what your goals are and stick to them. This will make you feel a lot more certain about who you are and where you're going.

4 Fake it till you make it. Look the part and after a while you'll start feeling the part. It's massively confidence building!

5 Learn to accept compliments. If people are saying nice things about you, chances are, they're true. So remember to believe them!

6 Eat healthily and allow yourself a few little treats – this will make you feel good about your body as well as making sure you get to indulge every now and again.

7 Exercise regularly – this is great for banishing worries and making sure you sleep well as well as keeping your figure firm.

 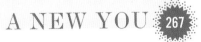

8 Get plenty of sleep. We all have such busy lives but clocking in at least eight hours of slumber keeps your skin looking peachy and makes sure you've got enough energy to keep up with the day.

9 Take risks – take a trip to that place you've always wanted to visit, try out that new class at the gym or buy that hot guy a drink in the bar. The looks of admiration and envy you'll get from your friends are enough to make you feel good about yourself!

10 Believe in yourself. A lot of life is a self-fulfilling prophecy, so if you believe that you can achieve that killer bod/bag that dream job/pull off those hot pants, the chances are you'll be able to.

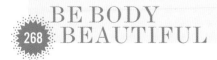

How to Wear the Right Clothes for Your Body Shape

One of my big annoyances is when girls say they can't find anything to wear for their shape. There is something for all shapes on the high street and you can look good no matter your size – you just need to spend some time working out what suits your figure and accentuates the best bits.

If you are over a size 12, I'd opt for pencil skirts, nipped in at the waist, and don't be afraid for things to hug your figure. Often people fall into the trap of wearing baggy clothes and that can make you look bigger than you actually are. Hourglass bodies and curves are beautiful. That said, I get very frustrated by people who are pro being plus-sized. It's not anything to do with being size-ist, it's about health. I firmly believe it is unhealthy to be carrying too much weight and when that's glorified by the media it is completely irresponsible to young girls and boys. I'd love to see healthy food and fitness properly implemented in schools and to help with that is one of my dreams left to accomplish. But ... getting back to dressing for your size!

Everyone has a part of their body or a problem area that they don't like very much – for instance, I don't like my legs particularly. I don't have the longest legs in the world so to accentuate them I like to wear a high heel and nudes always make your legs look longer. But don't forget to experiment with bright colours too, because they make you feel good and there are loads of options. And if you have short legs avoid shoes with a strap around the ankles, as they will make you look even shorter.

Always accentuate your best bits. If you have a flabby tummy, wear loosely fitted cami tops. Don't highlight your belly with a tight T-shirt that leaves nothing to the imagination! If your boobs are big don't flatten them; wear sculpted tops that make them look even better. And if you have a big bum then show it off like Kim and Beyoncé. Big bums are now cool! I love the one I got on *Tumble*. But unless you keep up the exercises it doesn't last!

 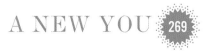

It's important to make fashion work for you. It can be tempting to try and work the latest trend no matter what your body shape is, but you'll end up looking much sexier if you stay true to yourself and show off your individual assets – be they your tiny waist, your slender pins, your fabulous cleavage or even your toned shoulders. No one look works for everyone, which is why I've decided to tailor my fashion tips to specific body types. There's something here that will make every woman look the best she can as well as being up to the minute.

Want to Look Slimmer? Here's How to Dress Slim

Whether you're a naturally curvy girl or have just piled on a few pounds recently, there's always a way to make the most of your voluptuousness and draw attention away from the bits you don't feel so confident about. It might surprise you that whether you're eight stone or twelve stone, your waist is almost always your narrowest part, so showcasing it is the number one rule of flattering the fuller figure. The quickest and easiest way to do this is by cinching it in with a stunning belt. Choose a darker-coloured belt than the rest of your outfit for the real Betty Boop factor.

The next fail-safe style tip for curvier girls is making sure that your clothes fit you properly. If you're not feeling very confident about your shape, it can be tempting to cover it up in big, baggy clothes. But far from skimming your shape, these tenty choices often just make you look much chunkier than you actually are.

The same goes for clothes that are too small. We've all been there: standing in changing rooms telling ourselves that we'll lose weight and buy the size 10, rather than admit we need the size 12. The thing is, as we all know, it's a waste of money as well as a disservice to your figure. Squeezing yourself into clothes that are a bit on the tight side won't make you look better. In fact, a too-small purchase will just showcase all of your lumps and bumps until you realize that you don't feel confident in it and that £40 piece of material is banished to the back of your wardrobe forevermore. Being honest with yourself and working with your figure while you get it to where you really want it is the best way of looking your sexiest.

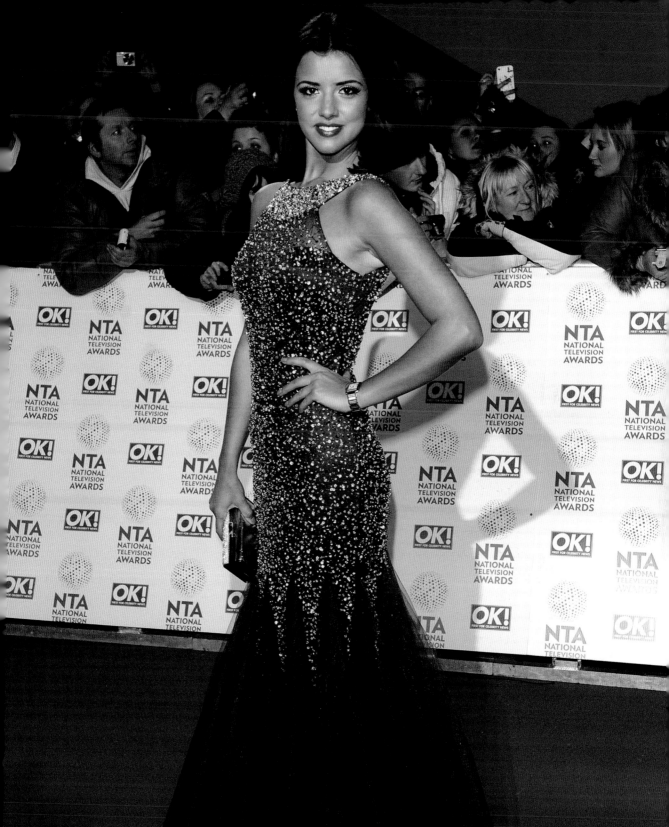

I've already told you that my legs are my least favourite part of my body but I can't lengthen them so I use fashion as a tool to make them look longer than they are. Lengthening your legs by wearing heels is also the cheat's way to a slimmer-looking figure. If they make your feet hurt at parties, don't panic. Just take them off after everyone's had a few. They'll only remember your fabulous first entrance! That said, fashion was never supposed to be comfortable. Work those heels, ladies!

Big Boobs? Small Boobs? Dress Them Right

If you're blessed with a great pair, don't spend all of your time trying to hide them in baggy T-shirts. Yes, big boobs can be a pain when you're bikini shopping or trying to pull off that backless dress, but they're ultimately the envy of other women and ooze pulling potential! You just need to remember how to make the most of them. This doesn't necessarily mean you need to put them – as my mum used to say – on a plate for everyone to see. It does mean, though, they need proper support.

Having your boobs lolling over your waistline because of an ill-fitting bra is not the most flattering look and can cheapen the style you're going for. I know it's sometimes hard to find affordable, well-fitting lingerie if you're particularly well endowed, but stores like Boux Avenue or Bravissimo offer DD+ bras that won't make you wince when you check your bank balance. I also love Gossard bras because they're so pretty and girly but are also properly made.

The beach can also be a nightmarish prospect for big-busted girls, but once you accept that string bikinis really aren't going to cut it for you, most of your problems are behind you. Make sure to also avoid any styles with ruffles in them, which will just make your boobs look even bigger.

Last but not least, no matter how fashionable drop-waist dresses and billowing, straight-down numbers are at the moment, they do no favours for the ample décolletage. Don't be tempted by how smart that smock looks on your flat-chested colleague – boobs and

BE BODY
BEAUTIFUL

baggy just don't mix. Instead, go for something that nips in your waist to leave everyone in no doubt of your curvilicious figure.

For the smaller ladies there are also loads of options on the market to make them perkier! Plenty of my mates have had breast implants and I'm not the greatest fan – they need a lot of upkeep and they do look very fake! You can get some good implants that are made to look far more natural but they still don't have a look that I particularly like. Gel bras, push-up bras and good old chicken fillets can often achieve the same look. Plus smaller-breasted women can own those string bikinis and backless dresses! And, besides, it's really fashionable to have small boobs. Look at Kate Moss, Kendall Jenner, Cara Delevingne – they don't have big boobs. There are positives to everything!

What to Wear if you Want a Few More Curves

Our society tends to assume that life's a breeze for skinny people. But being naturally slim can have its problems just as much as for any other figure. When I was at my smallest I used clothes to my advantage. I often went for fabrics with lots of patterns on them but in pale shades. These really soften out your body. I also made the most of being able to wear the coolest fashion trends – like smock dresses, hot pants and crop tops. They gave me back my sense of fun and encouraged me to exercise to stay on top of my shape rather than deprive myself food-wise.

Everyone has 'Fat' Days, Right?

I'm pretty sure that every woman wakes up and just feels rubbish every now and again. It might be because you're on your period, or you might have been really busy at work and not had time to exercise as much as usual. You might have just got too excited about that takeaway the night before. Regardless of the reason, I've got a few fall-back plans to deal with that.

Start the day with a green tea and end the day with one too. And make sure you drink your two litres of water. (In fact, you should

 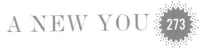

do that every day – at first you will wee a lot but your body soon gets used to it and your skin will feel better almost instantly.) Peppermint tea is a good digestive and helps after a meal.

On THOSE days I dress in one of my favourite, easy outfits, something that I'm not going to have to fuss over all day. Don't go to the extreme and put on something really baggy, though, because that can often have the opposite effect and make you feel even bigger. I also make sure that I do my make-up extra specially and wear some fabulous earrings. Then no one will look at your body – they'll just be captivated by your face!

My Style Rules

I stick by a few rules when it comes to fashion.

Number one: I'm not a stranger to showing off flesh but I like to keep it classy. If I'm wearing a low-cut top, I try to team it with slim jeans or a maxi skirt. Or if I want to wear hot pants or a short skirt, I'll wear something high-necked on top.

I apply the same principle to make-up. If I wear a vampy lipstick, I usually make sure my eyes are as natural as possible, with only a few sweeps of a neutral shade of eyeshadow.

I also firmly believe that less is more. This goes both for my face and my clothes. We all have old pictures that we look back on and hate. They scream: TOO MUCH bronzer or TOO MUCH blusher! I do like wearing high fashion but I don't like anything too fussy. I like classic looks that make you look sleek and glamorous.

One thing my mum always used to tell me is to try things on. You might think something looks hideous on the hanger but it can actually be transformed when you're wearing it. Or vice versa. And trying on one extra dress whenever you go shopping isn't really that much work, is it?

High heels are key and when you're going out just take a small clutch so it's impossible to take too much out with you. Only carry a big bag if you're having a 'fat' day and hold it across your tummy.

BE BODY
BEAUTIFUL

A staple black blazer is a must-have for any wardrobe. Try and get one that's structured and tailored. Invest a bit more in it because it will stay in your wardrobe for years to dress up everything from jeans and a T-shirt to shorts and a cami or a little dress.

Accept that if something doesn't suit you then it doesn't suit you. It's better to wear things that flatter your figure than be a die-hard fashionista. For example, I love culottes but I can't wear them. I wish I could, but they look terrible on me, so I won't go near them!

Hairstyles Make a BIG Difference to Your Look

I love changing my hair every now and then. It makes me feel good and keeps things current and fresh. I never thought I'd cut my long hair but in a weird way it was one of the best things I ever did! I love it short, although it's harder to manage and I get occasional hair envy when I see girls with longer hair! So it's good to mix it up. Shorter is definitely harder to manage though . . . Always keep some extensions in your hair collection and there are some fab hairpieces on the market in case you really want to change your look for a night or your short hair isn't behaving as it should do! Hair is the first thing to look bad when you're feeling a bit rubbish or under the weather, so hair extensions and hairpieces can be a real lifesaver. And besides, it can be so much fun to change your look instantly without waiting several months for your hair to grow or having to go to the hairdressers.

Don't over-wash your hair – it doesn't need washing every day. You can always pop a bit of dry shampoo in if you really think you need it but don't use that too often either because it can dry your hair out. Styling hair is a lot easier when you haven't washed it that day.

Always, always keep a comb and a mini hairspray in your bag when you go out. When I'm out with my mates I inevitably pop to the ladies and fix my hair – especially after having a dance. If you've got an up-do it'll always slip a bit. And having voluminous hair always makes your face look better.

 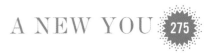

The most important thing to remember about hair, though, is to take as good care of it as possible and protect it from all of the styling products you use. Dry, frazzled hair looks horrible so make sure you look after your hair, especially if you dye it. Use a conditioning treatment whenever possible.

Make-up Dos and Don'ts

As I get older I think I am getting much better at doing my own make-up. But it really is a case of practice makes perfect.

One mistake girls often make is to never vary their look. Experiment with different styles when you have a bit of time because make-up can change your appearance dramatically and make a real statement. I love trying out different looks and testing new make-up trends. But I'm always careful to make sure that I use products that accentuate rather than hide my features. There's nothing worse than seeing people wear foundation like a mask, seeing the line under their chin where the foundation stops and the neck begins. It looks cheap and tacky.

I always use a good brush (I have a Bobbi Brown one) to apply my foundation and I never wear the same foundation tone in winter as I do in summer. For the winter you need a warmer tone and for the summer a darker but fresher one, because skin is much more tanned than in winter. I use Giorgio Armani's luminous silk foundation.

Spend time on your eye make-up, opening them up. For a night out you can afford to wear really heavy make-up. A great tip to remember is to apply white eyeliner inside the rims of your eyes. It makes your eyes appear bigger and brighter, even though you wouldn't think it!

The number one rule of make-up is to use well-selected products. I don't necessarily mean expensive products, just ones that you know work. Often it is the more expensive products that do work best, but it's still a good idea to save for them because in the long run they last longer anyway as you don't have to re-apply them every five minutes. Cheaper products can sometimes be a false economy.

And if you're going to wear fake eyelashes, don't forget to take the glue out with you – there's nothing worse than a girl walking around with half an eyelash hanging off.

⊙•⦿•⊙•⊙•⦿•⊙

On the subject of skin, I can't stress how important it is to make sure you remove your make-up before you go to bed. It's so tempting to flop down when you get in after a night out and not bother taking it off but that does a lot of damage. In Essex loads of girls love fake tan and I love to have a bit of colour too, but when I was doing *Tumble* I had to wear more fake tan than normal, and also much more make-up, to look good under the performance lights. As soon as it was over and I got home I would take all the make-up off, otherwise my skin would be dry and spotty. There's nothing worse than waking up with your pores feeling all blocked up and your mascara all over your cheeks.

Face wipes are an easy way to remove your make-up and work really well. I use Dermalogica eye make-up remover and Simple make-up wipes but you shouldn't use make-up wipes every day, as they don't get everything off your face. You need to cleanse, tone and moisturize too (as many days as possible), which I know is the last thing you want to do when you're tired and you just want to jump into bed. I do that at least three times a week to make sure my pores are completely clean. Exfoliation is important too – I use an Elemis product to exfoliate my skin and take off all the dead skin. It gives my skin a really healthy glow instantly, then I moisturize with Elizabeth Arden moisturizing cream. Exfoliate your body too. If you are a fan of fake tan it's the only way to stop the tan going streaky when you apply it and the only way to get it to stay on for longer. The simpler you make your skincare regime, the more likely you are to stick to it, but do try to exfoliate your face and body at least once a week to keep your skin fresh and smooth.

You'll already know that nutrition is key in keeping your skin peachy and eating healthily has a knock-on effect on your hair and nails too. Eating nutrient-rich foods like avocado and salmon is a great way to replenish your skin, hair and nails. Try having half an avocado with your breakfast every day to see real results.

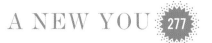

MY TOP TEN MAKE-UP BAG MUST-HAVES

1 Giorgio Armani Luminous Silk Foundation – it makes your skin glow and is light enough to let your natural skin shine through.

2 MAC Prep + Prime Transparent Finishing Powder

3 My favourite mascara: Maybelline Volum' Express The Colossal Mascara

4 MAC Lip Pencil in Spice – I love vampy colours and this pencil creates glamour without looking too extreme.

5 My eyebrows are tattooed by Tracie Giles but I also like to go over them in the mornings with HD Eye & Brow Palette. Strong eyebrows are really striking and instantly make your face look better. When I was younger I used to pluck them until they were really thin, like everyone else at school. Now I like to keep them thicker.

6 I love to be bronzed and use Sunkissed Gradual Tanning Lotion – it gives a really healthy natural tan. And when you want a bit of a holiday glow, try YSL Terre Saharienne Bronzing Powder – it's just gorgeous.

7 Dior 5 Couleurs Eyeshadow Palette in Femme-Fleur – but there are so many colours in the palettes that I love. You can mix and match depending on the occasion.

BE BODY BEAUTIFUL

8 YSL Touche Éclat – for those days when you want your eyes to hide a late night before!

9 L'Oréal Paris Infallible Eyeliner in Night Day Black – it lasts for hours and gives a lovely mix of somewhere in between kohl and liquid.

10 Eylure Volume 107 Lashes – never be without a spare set of false eyelashes because you never know when your peepers need a little awakening. And remember that less is often more, so don't overdo it, just find a style that suits your eye shape.

Getting Ready for a Night Out

The night before, remember to apply your fake tan so you're nice and bronzed. Then on the night you're going out make sure you moisturize.

Always start early – the last thing you want to be doing is rushing because nothing ever goes right. First off I have a shower and put on a dressing gown. The girls will come round and we'll pour a glass of wine and put some music on. What should take half an hour then takes about four hours! On the nights I am going out I try and pop to the hairdressers during the day for a blow-dry so that I can concentrate on doing my make-up. Once I'm all made-up I put my clothes on. They are the last thing to go on before I head out because I don't want to spill anything on them or get them creased.

Getting ready for a night out should be fun. I love getting properly glammed up with a few of my best mates, like Kayleigh, Abi, Keeley and Monica. We have such a laugh when we are getting ready and it makes the evening feel longer.

TOP BEAUTY TIPS

1   If you have short legs avoid shoes with a strap around the ankles, as they will make you look even shorter.

2   Exfoliate your face and body at least once a week to keep your skin fresh and smooth.

3   Try and get eight hours' sleep a night. It's good for your skin and your mind.

4   Start the day with a green tea and end it with one too. In between, drink two litres of water.

5   Most importantly – ENJOY life, but be healthy and enjoy it for longer.

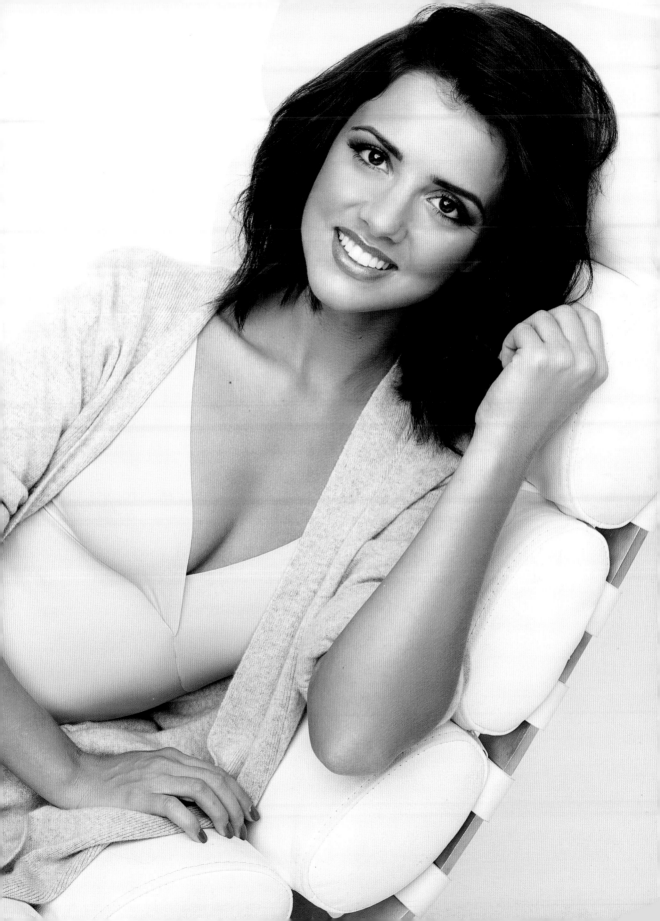

Acknowledgements

Firstly, a big thank you to everyone who has helped me be me. Who'd have thought that Lucy Mecklenburgh from Essex would be where I am today? How exciting. It's already been an amazing journey and I can't thank my family and friends enough for the huge amount of support they've given me over the years. I wouldn't be where I am without you.

Without my mum and dad I definitely wouldn't have been able to take the opportunities I have. They always stand by me, always give me their honest advice, make me roast dinners and fix my washing machine!

Thank you to Scarlett Short, my fabulous agent and publicist, who has stood by me through some of the hardest times of my life and believed in me when even I didn't. You've helped me achieve things I could never have imagined and, most importantly, you're a friend for life. Thank you.

To Kirsty Reilly, my super-fun modelling agent – thank you for helping me play the biggest game of dress-up ever and for all our hilarious work trips.

Cecilia and Frank Harris have helped me massively with our business and I can't thank them enough for their help – it's been amazingly successful and I'm very proud of what we have achieved. Cecilia – you helped me transform my body and that has been life-changing.

Emma Whitnall, the woman who swapped my diet from McDonalds to fruit smoothies and breakfast roughies! You've done what I thought no one could for my digestion! You've re-educated me and transformed the way I look.

Finally, thank you to Hannah Fernando, my unbelievably patient ghost writer who listened to my stories until 2am and made them sound exactly how I wanted, and to the lovely Fenella Bates at Penguin, who believed in me enough to commission this book. It's always been a dream and I'm one lucky girl.

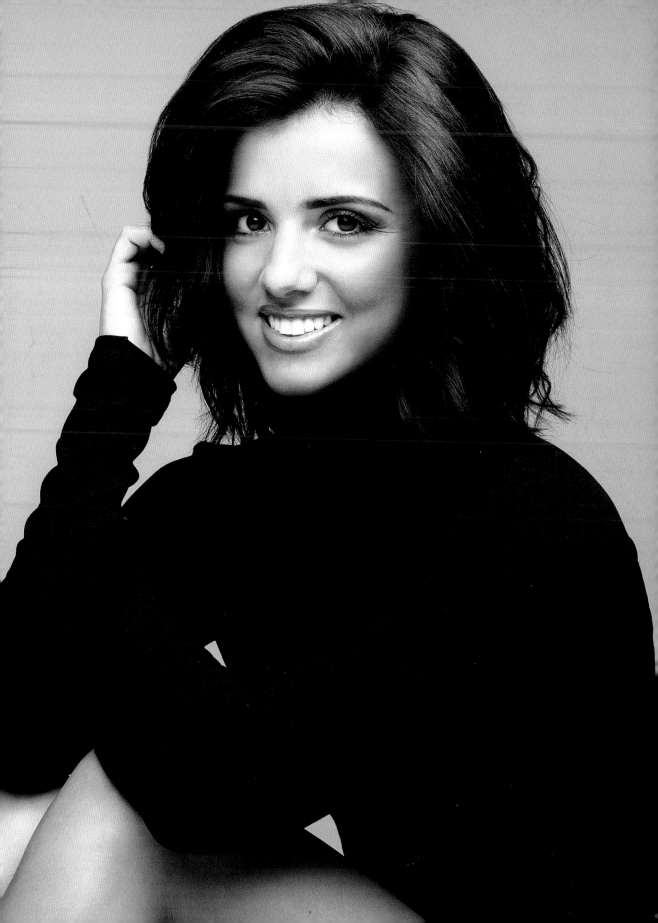

Image Permissions

Principal photography © Catherine Harbour: cover image, and pages 2, 6, 32, 36, 42, 53, 73, 107, 108, 111, 138, 150, 242, 249, 252, 257, 263, 280-81

Photography by Isabella Haigh and food styling by Hanna Hill: pages 168, 169, 172, 191, 199, 204, 208, 210, 213, 214, 216, 219

Additional images copyright:

© **Lucy Mecklenburgh and family:** pages 14, 15, 122

© **Results with Lucy:** pages 120, 122, 125, 126, 128, 131, 145, 149, 224, 232, 235, 236, 241

© **Results with Bump:** page 46

© **Marbella Photo/Rex:** pages 24, 39

© **Xposurephotos.com:** page 270

© **Poisson D'avnl/Photocuisine:** page 49

© **Food & Drink/Photocuisine:** page 51

© **Stockfood/Rua Castilho:** page 64

© **Thys/Supperdelux/Photocuisine:** page 67

© **Court/Photocuisine:** pages 69, 92, 160

© **Gelberger/Photocuisine:** page 77

© **Stockfood/Olga Miltsova:** pages 82, 180

© **Stockfood/Clive Streeter:** page 90

© **Stockfood/Lars Ranek:** pages 95, 155, 157

© **Cultura Creative/Photocuisine:** pages 102, 165, 166

© **BBC Photo Library:** page 116

© **Carnet/Photocuisine:** page 153

© **Fénot/Photocuisine:** page 159

© **Stockfood/Food & Drink Photos/Jemma Watts:** page 179

© **Stockfood/Bernhard Winkleman:** page 183

© **Amiel/Photocuisine:** page 185

© **Leser/Photocuisine:** page 188

© **Stockfood/David Loftus:** page 196

© **Sudres/Photocuisine:** page 223

© **Ellesse:** page 133, 149

© **Sunkissed:** pages 22, 245

With thanks to Claire, Jessica, Katie, Laura, Laura and Louise for their before-and-after photos.

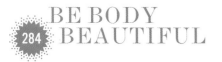

RECIPE NOTES

RECIPE NOTES

EXERCISE NOTES

GET RESULTS WITH LUCY

EXCLUSIVE READER DISCOUNT OF 20% OFF A SUBSCRIPTION TO THE RESULTS WITH LUCY WEBSITE.*

GO TO:
WWW.RESULTSWITHLUCY.COM/
BEBODYBEAUTIFUL

*OFFER ENDS 31ST JANUARY 2016.
FOR TERMS AND CONDITIONS, VISIT
WWW.RESULTSWITHLUCY.COM/
BEBODYBEAUTIFUL